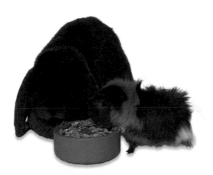

Natural Healthcare for Pets

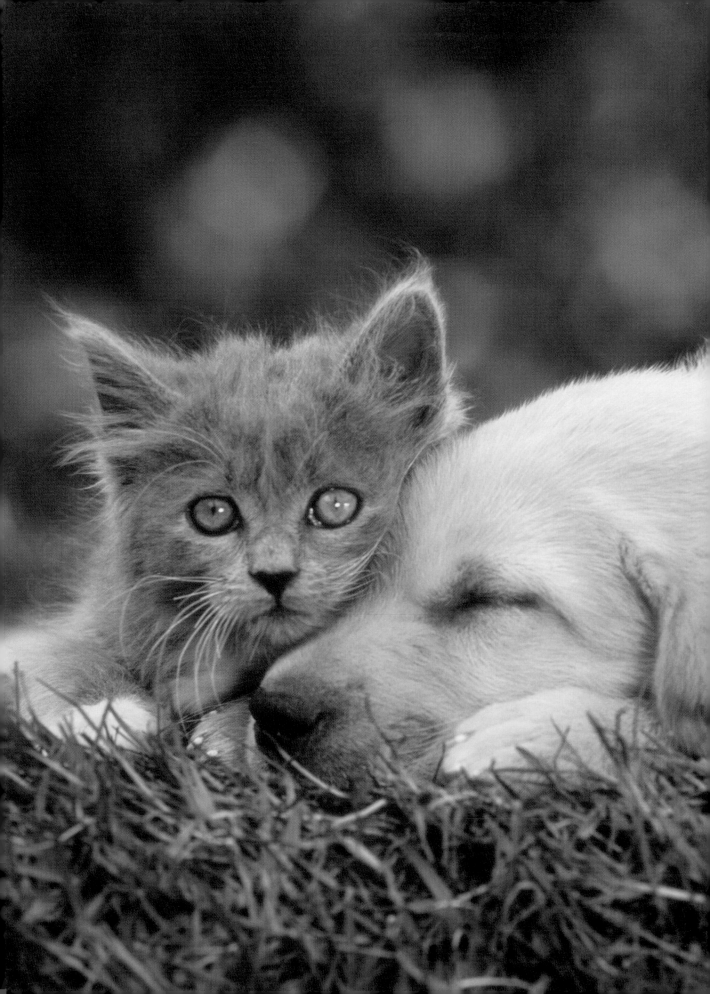

Natural Healthcare for Pets

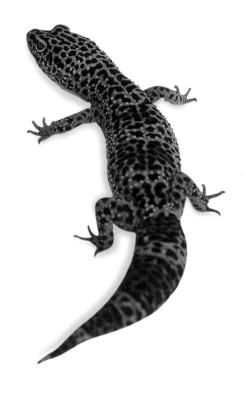

Richard Allport

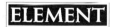

For my sons Julian and Josh, whom I love dearly.
"We have seen, and split, the atom
But true love is invisible, indivisible."
Thanks to Wendie Bowen for spinning this web of words from my spidery handwriting.

Element
An Imprint of HarperCollins*Publishers*
77–85 Fulham Palace Road
Hammersmith, London W6 8JB

Element™ is a trademark of HarperCollins*Publishers* Limited

First published in Great Britain in 2001 by
Element Books Limited

2 4 6 8 10 9 7 5 3 1

Text copyright © Richard Allport
Copyright © HarperCollins*Publishers* Ltd

Richard Allport asserts the moral right to
be identified as the author of this work

A catalog record for this book
is available from the British Library

ISBN 0 00 713087 2

Printed and bound in Italy

This book was designed and produced by
HE BRIDGEWATER BOOK COMPANY

CREATIVE DIRECTOR Terry Jeavons
EDITORIAL DIRECTOR Fiona Biggs
DESIGNER Colin Fielder
PROJECT EDITOR Lizzy Gray
PICTURE RESEARCHER Lynda Marshall
PHOTOGRAPHER Marc Henrie

Disclaimer

This book is not able to replace your veterinarian. It is a guide to natural ways of keeping pets healthy
and helping them when they are ill. Whenever acute or persistent symptoms of illness occur, consult
your veterinarian. Never risk your pets' health by delaying a visit to the veterinarian. The remedies
listed in the following pages are normally safe when used as instructed. However, any remedy, even a
natural medicine, may cause an unusual reaction in an occasional individual. If any unexpected effect
seems to be caused by any remedy, consult your veterinarian immediately.

Contents

Introduction

It may be thought that there is no need for a book on natural healthcare for domestic animals. It seems that pets are living longer and more comfortably than they were a few decades ago. Modern pharmaceutical drugs cope with disease, pet food manufacturers produce a wide variety of foods, and pets are usually housed in our warm homes. But look a little closer. If food, housing, and modern drugs are so wonderful, why is there so much chronic physical and mental illness in pets?

The reality is that many modern pet foods contain additives that are unnecessary at best, or potentially harmful at worst. Some ingredients are of questionable origin and dental disease is rife among cats and dogs fed on soft canned food.

Our homes are hermetically sealed, centrally heated, or air-conditioned. Lack of fresh air and sunlight contributes to poor physical health, and lack of exercise, and social interaction leads to poor mental health.

Modern drugs may treat acute diseases effectively, but often have no real answer to many chronic diseases. Use of drugs such as antibiotics and steroids can suppress disease rather than cure it. And the drugs themselves frequently have side-effects, which can seriously weaken the immune system and result in even more health problems.

This book shows you how to keep your pet in the healthiest condition possible. It gives advice on a healthy lifestyle, natural and nutritious diets, supplements to boost the immune system and reduce illness, and safe, natural remedies for ailments.

There are four sections: a healthy lifestyle; natural therapies and using them; common pet diseases and how to treat them; and the final section – first aid for pets as well, as how to cope with saying goodbye.

Natural Healthcare for Pets contains advice on the care of all common domestic pets; these include – dogs, cats, guinea pigs, hamsters, ferrets, birds, fish, chelonians, and reptiles.

The healthy lifestyle section is a guide to promoting and maintaining good health – both physical and mental. It gives advice on basic nutrition as well as supplements to boost the immune system; how to keep your pet well-housed and comfortable; ways to avoid the effects of chemicals and other pollutants in the environment; and tips on keeping your pet's mind, as well as body, active.

The therapies covered include all the useful and effective natural treatments for pets. From acupuncture, aromatherapy, and flower remedies, to crystals, homeopathy, herbs and massage techniques, as well as nutritional advice. Some of these therapies must be left to the experts to practice; it isn't recommended to try acupuncture yourself, for example. Others, such as gem remedies, are safe for you to give to your pet following the instructions here.

The disease section includes all the common ailments which pets are likely to encounter. To make it easier to use, diseases of various parts of the body are grouped together, so that skin problems are in one section, digestive tract conditions in another, and so on. There are special sections on parasites, specific bacteria, viruses and cancer. Another section covers mental problems – from aggression and anxiety to eating disorders and depression. For each of these diseases there is a list of natural, safe and effective remedies which can help to relieve symptoms and promote healing.

The final section covers first aid treatment using natural remedies for accidents, injuries, and other emergencies. It also deals with that all too important time – saying goodbye.

ABOVE Many manufactured pet foods contain unnecessary and potentially harmful additives.

OPPOSITE To ensure its good health, do not let your dog become a couch potato.

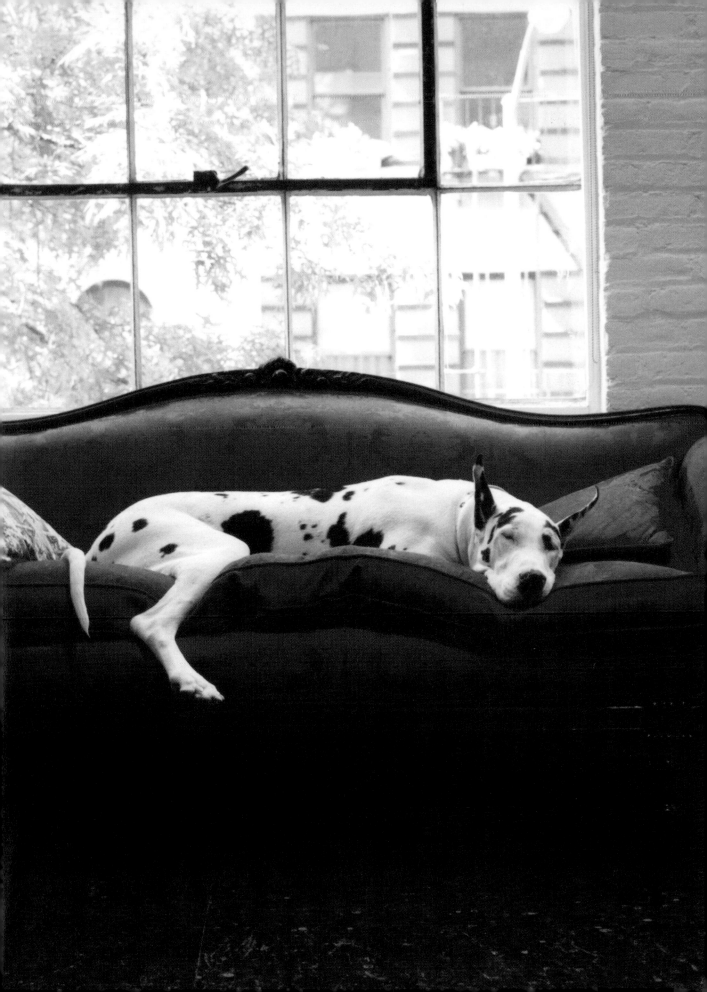

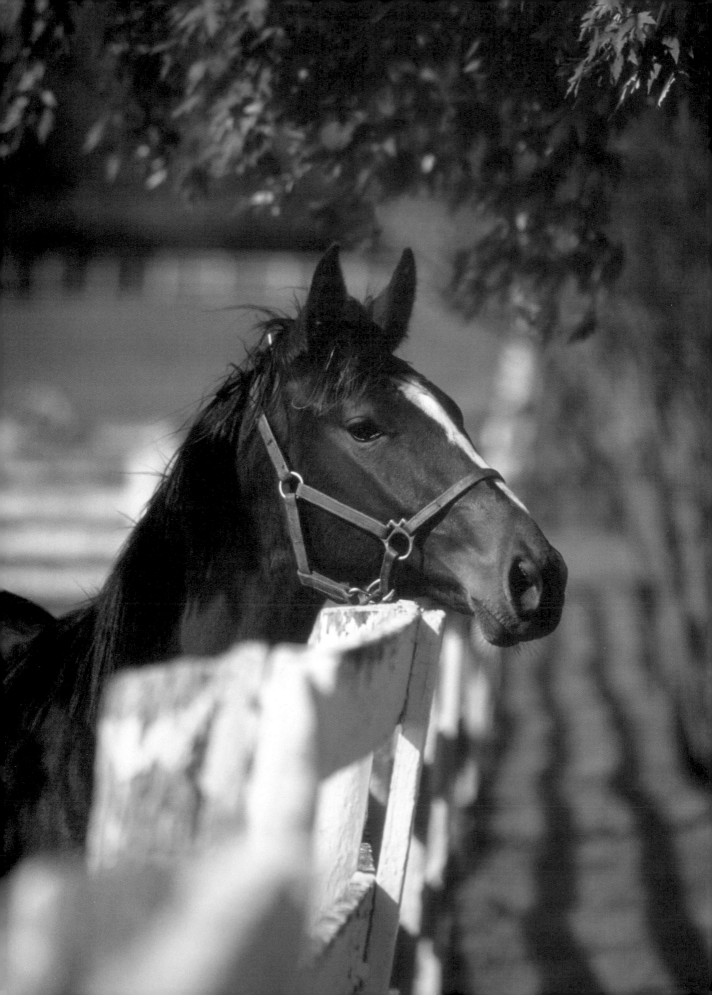

Part I

A Healthy Lifestyle

A healthy lifestyle means thinking about diet and nutrition, supplements to enhance health and boost the immune system, providing the best environment for your pet, minimizing the effects of pollution, and keeping pets healthy mentally as well as physically.

A HEALTHY BODY

As far as possible, diet should provide foods that are closest to the natural diet of the pet concerned. We are what we eat, and so are our pets; optimal nutrition is vital to pet health. Many pet foods, especially canned foods, contain artificial colorings, flavorings, preservatives, and other additives, as well as unacceptably high levels of salt, and even sugar – especially in pet treats. Depending on supplies used, pet foods may have been stored for too long or in unhygienic conditions. Molds, which can be toxic, sometimes grow in hay stored for rabbits and other small pets, and mice and rats may gain access to stored pet food. Try and ensure that commercially prepared food is of the best quality, with the fewest additives, and from a reliable supplier.

Many pet foods claim to contain a perfectly balanced mix of nutrients – but if the stress and pollution in our daily lives means we may need extra supplements added to our diets, the same applies to our pets. Supplements will support the immune system and help prevent illness.

The home environment is not necessarily all it could be. Goldfish are still kept in bowls, rabbits in cramped hutches, and birds in tiny cages, while dogs are chained up all day. Pets need an appropriate amount of space, at the right temperature and the right humidity – not just to be well fed and watered.

A HEALTHY MIND

And finally, it is important to keep pets healthy mentally. Animals need to be stimulated mentally; admittedly, some more than others. There are few sadder sights than a budgerigar in a bare cage, with nothing to do and no companion.

Maintaining a healthy lifestyle is probably the most important section in this book. Pets that have good nutrition, a strong immune system, minimal exposure to pollutants and other immune damaging substances, have appropriate housing and exercise facilities, and are mentally and physically fit and active undoubtedly stand much less risk of contracting disease.

In fact if you follow the advice in the healthy lifestyle for pets section, your own health will benefit too!

Nutrition

Environment

Mental well-being

A healthy lifestyle and environment is essential to maintain healthy animals.

Diet

If you feed your pet entirely on canned and dried foods, you will certainly not be starving it. However, nor will you be providing it with an optimum diet that will ensure it maintains good health and energy levels as well as happiness. To be fit and healthy, the diet should be as natural as possible. And ideally, this should be as close as possible to the normal foods that would be eaten in the wild. Don't feel bad if you open a can of petfood, but make sure that it contains the best ingredients available. Think about what natural foods you can add to the basic diet to make it both more interesting and more healthy. Elderly and pregnant pets, working animals, and young, growing pets may have different requirements from the following general dietary advice. For such animals, always consult your veterinarian before varying the diet.

WEIGHT

Never change a pet's diet suddenly; introduce any changes gradually over a period of weeks. If in doubt, consult your veterinarian. There is no fixed amount of food any one type of pet needs – age, breed, size, amount of exercise, and normal metabolic rate, all affect the quantity. But do not let your pet get overweight – there are too many associated problems.

Keep a check on the weight of your pet.

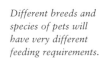

Different breeds and species of pets will have very different feeding requirements.

FEEDING YOUR DOG

Dogs are omnivores with a bias toward carnivorousness. It is quite feasible to provide a vegetarian diet; this can relieve allergies and bowel disorders. However, in the wild, dogs eat meat, and this should be part of their diet.

MEAT
• 40 percent raw meat, preferably organic.
• Feed meat in chunks to let your dog chew well.
• Do not feed red meat only, but include fish and poultry.
• Raw chicken wings are an ideal basic meat source.
• Include heart, tripe, kidneys, and small amounts of liver.
• Big, juicy marrow bones are good sources of calcium and roughage – and help clean teeth.

OTHER INGREDIENTS
• 60 percent of diet should be vegetables, fruit, grains and pulses (whole-wheat bread, cooked brown rice, chopped nuts, diced or grated raw vegetables, and non-citrus fruits).

• Eggs are nutritious, but no more than one or two per week. Give one or two teaspoons of live yogurt daily.
• Milk is acceptable in small amounts and is a good source of calcium, but some dogs cannot digest milk.
• Oils: natural oils such as sesame, sunflower, and safflower oil help keep skin and coat glossy and in good condition. Give one teaspoon twice weekly.

TREATS
Avoid chocolate, or anything fattening. Most proprietary treats contain sugars – so be sure to choose the sugar-free ones. Dried liver and garlic make tasty treats that most dogs adore. Available in tablets, or cook your own.

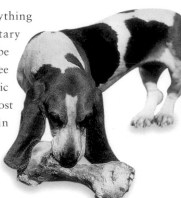

Fresh bones for chewing are essential to a healthy diet.

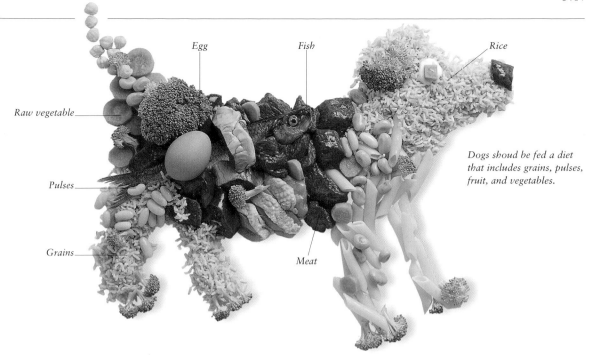

Egg

Fish

Rice

Raw vegetable

Pulses

Grains

Meat

Dogs shoud be fed a diet that includes grains, pulses, fruit, and vegetables.

FEEDING YOUR CAT

Cats are obligate carnivores and so cannot be vegetarian. There are two nutrients that cats need to stay healthy, which are found only in animal tissue: arachadonic acid, one of the essential fatty acids and needed for healthy skin, kidneys, and reproduction; and taurine, an amino acid, needed for normal retinal function of the eyes. A deficiency of taurine causes blindness.

Cats are notoriously fussy, demanding that their food is as tasty and fresh as possible. In the wild, they will kill and eat mice, voles, small rabbits, and birds. This provides them with the minerals, vitamins, fiber, and carbohydrate to balance the protein in the muscle meat of their prey. The internal organs contain partly digested grains and other vegetable matter, which cats need for balanced nourishment.

Cats that hunt can feed themselves, but this is not necessarily to be encouraged. Provide your cat with the following diet, and the need to hunt should be diminished.

MEAT

• Should be about 60 percent of diet, and raw meat is preferable, organic if possible.
• Include fish and poultry – giving red meat only will overload the digestion of many domestic cats.
• Cooking destroys some nutrients, but rabbit and pork should not be given raw, as they may contain parasites.
• Give meat in chunks that are large enough to make your cat chew – this is good for teeth and jaws.

• Offal – heart, tripe, kidneys, and a little liver should always be included.
• Liver fed in large amounts will cause an overdose of vitamin A, so give small amounts only.

OTHER INGREDIENTS

• Should be about 40 percent of diet and include vegetables, fruit, grains, and pulses (cooked brown rice, grated carrots and zucchini, corn, and unsweetened cereals).
• Grains and pulses should be cooked, not raw.
• Eggs are nutritious – no more than one or two a week.
• Live yogurt is high in both nutrients and natural bacteria that helps efficient digestion.
• Milk is suitable for most cats in small amounts, but some cats have a milk allergy, which may cause diarrhea.
• Oils such as sesame, sunflower, and safflower improve skin and coat condition – give one teaspoon.

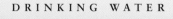

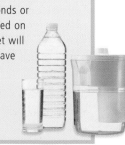

DRINKING WATER

Give filtered or mineral water, not tap water. Cats often drink little from the bowl provided, but prefer to drink from ponds or puddles outside. Cats fed on a mainly dried food diet will drink more and must have fresh water available at all times.

Always provide a bowl of fresh mineral water.

PET BIRDS

All birds need at least six different food items in their diet. Because of this need for variety, it is often preferable to feed proprietary, pre-packed bird foods as a basic diet. To this should be added:

• Green foods – lettuce, watercress, chickweed, parsley, dandelion.

• Vegetables – sprouted seeds, carrots, beet.

• Fruits – oranges, apples, plums, grapes.

• For preference, these foods should be organic. If not, wash thoroughly before use.

• Seed-eating birds need grit to help digest their food. Include oyster shell, eggshell, and quartz in the grit.

• Birds other than parrots, budgies, canaries, and finches will have different requirements. Consult your vet.

• Water must be available at all times – filtered or mineral, change regularly.

Ensure a balanced diet by feeding your bird fresh vegetable leaves and roots, as well as fruits and a proprietary bird food.

nutritious foods to make the diet as healthy as possible. Fresh and clean, mineral or filtered water should be available at all times. Any added fresh foods, such as vegetables, fruits, hay, or seeds should be washed before use, and should not have been treated with insecticides or herbicides.

CHINCHILLAS

Feed rabbit or guinea pig mix. Add good quality clover hay, carrots, cut grass, and green vegetables.

GERBILS

Feed rat or mouse food mix. Add some green leafy foods, such as cabbage or lettuce, in small amounts.

Give a few sunflower seeds only – too many cause metabolic imbalance and bone damage.

Dried fish food can be fed as crumbs, flakes, or pellets.

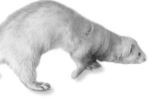

Ferrets need a diet that is high-protein, low-fat, and low-carbohydrate.

FERRETS

Ferrets are totally carnivorous. This often means that feeding a proprietary ferret food as a basic diet is most practicable. However, some raw meat should always be given – always make sure this is of good quality.

• Whole day-old chicks are ideal.

• A little milk is alright, but the "bread and milk" of folk tradition is not.

• Cat food is suitable.

• Ferrets need a high-protein, low-carbohydrate, low-fat diet.

• They normally gain some weight in the winter and lose it in the summer.

RABBITS, RODENTS, AND GUINEA PIGS

In general, the nutritional requirements of these pets make it more realistic to feed a proprietary food mix, adding natural,

GUINEA PIGS

Feed a guinea pig mix. Add plenty of hay and green foods. Guinea pigs need lots of vitamin C, so add foods such as parsley, green peppers, sprouts, and broccoli, which are rich in vitamin C.

HAMSTERS

Feed a hamster mix. Add seeds, grains, fruits, and vegetables. Make sure all food is as fresh as possible; hamsters need more vitamins and minerals than most small pets.

RABBITS

Feed a balanced rabbit mix and provide hay and grass daily.

Rabbits should be fed a proprietary rabbit mix and a range of fresh leaves, vegetables, grass, and hay.

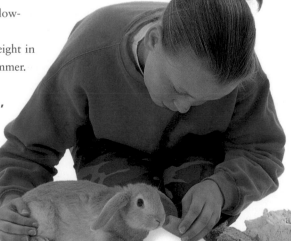

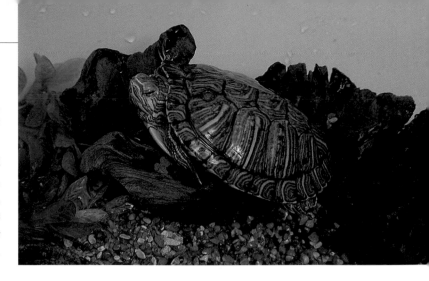

Terrapins are usually housed in a large tank or aquarium. They should be fed away from their main living area.

Feed a range of grain foods, vegetables, and garden weeds daily. For example, broccoli, cabbage and cauliflower leaves, ground elder, dandelions, and chickweed. Some rabbits produce red urine after eating dandelions or cabbage this is normal and no cause for concern.

RATS AND MICE

Feed rat/mouse mix. Add apples, tomatoes, and biscuits. Rats like sweet things. A little chocolate or cake is acceptable as an occasional treat or reward – but only occasionally!

FISH

A basic diet of proprietary pellet, flake, or crumb mix is usually more practicable for fish – but fish will be healthier and happier with some natural food too. Feed small earthworms – not those from a compost heap or from ground where herbicides or pesticides have been used. Fish are easily overfed. Roughly all that can be taken in two minutes twice a day is sufficient. If food is left at the bottom of the tank or pond, you are feeding too much.

TORTOISES

Tortoises are essentially vegetarian but do eat some meat in the wild – usually dead birds and mice. Most vegetables are suitable, but an excess of any one ingredient is best avoided since it may become poisonous. Fruits such as apples, pears, melons, strawberries, banana, and peaches are also suitable. Appropriate animal protein includes

Crickets, and locusts, along with plenty of vegetables, should be fed to reptiles.

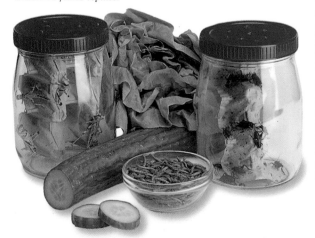

hard-cooked eggs and an occasional spoonful of canned cat or dog food. The American Box Tortoise is carnivorous and should be fed mealworms, slugs, snails, earthworms, and woodlice. They will eat fruit and vegetables too.

TERRAPINS

Terrapins are fish-eaters. They should be fed separately from their main living area, since they tend to leave uneaten food in their water, which will decompose and act as a pollutant. Feed sprats, herrings, shrimp, sardines, and pilchards. They will also eat tadpoles, water beetles, water snails, and earthworms. Growing terrapins need a piece of cuttlefish in the tank, since they are particularly prone to vitamin deficiency, which causes a distinctive white eye discharge. Providing cuttlefish (which are packed with vitamins) will ensure this deficiency does not occur.

LIZARDS AND SNAKES

Snakes are carnivorous, but need to be fed the correct type and size of small mammal. Consult an expert on what is suitable for the particular species you have and how often it should be fed. Some snakes eat fish or small lizards.
Lizards are more varied in their dietary requirements. Some eat insects, some are herbivorous, some are omnivorous – consult an expert on the correct diet. Always replicate the wild diet as closely as possible.

Lizards and snakes have different diets according to the species.

Supplements and the Immune System

A good, healthy, natural diet is important to keep the immune system functioning effectively, but if the diet doesn't consist totally of natural, organic, additive-free food, there are a range of supplements, manufactured specifically for animals, which will help.

VITAMINS AND MINERALS

Ideally, the best way to give vitamins and minerals is to feed foods that are rich in the particular supplement in question. In practice, it is difficult to ensure that sufficient vitamins and minerals are present in the diet. Supplements can be easily given in the form of a liquid, powder, or tablet versions. Here are a few tips on choosing correctly:

• Some vitamins are synthetic forms of the "natural" substance. Look for vitamin supplements which state "natural;" read the information on the packaging carefully and ask your supplier if you are not sure.

• The fewer extraneous filling and packing agents, the better. A long list of ingredients other than the actual vitamins and minerals is to be avoided.

• Buy vitamin and mineral supplements in small amounts. Despite a long expiry date, the contents of a pack do deteriorate once opened, especially in the case of vitamins. Don't buy in a five-year supply because of a special offer!

• Make sure the supplement comes in a form your pet will be able to take fairly easily; don't try to give huge tablets to a hamster!

Vitamins reduce skin ulceration in fish.

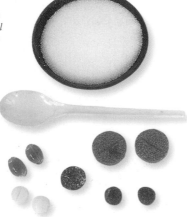

Supplements of vitamins and minerals are a useful method of insuring your pet has a nutritionally balanced diet.

POINTERS

• Water-soluble vitamins may leach out of fish pellets. Vitamin deficiency can cause some skin ulcerations on fish. An alternative method is to freeze liquid multivitamins in ice cube trays and then put one into the tank once a week for fish to nibble at.

• Cage birds particularly need vitamins A, D3, and B12 – these are found in so-called "conditioning" foods that are available for birds. Small amounts of these vitamins can be given as a supplement and mixed in with the ordinary diet.

• All tortoises and terrapins benefit from a multivitamin and mineral supplement, but it must be correctly balanced. Consult a vet on a suitable mixture for your pet.

Cage birds have specific vitamin needs.

Seek advice on a suitable vitamin and mineral supplement for tortoises.

• Hamsters have a particular need for vitamins and minerals because their digestion is different from other small rodents. They digest protein and carbohydrates more efficiently, but absorb fewer vitamins and minerals.

• Guinea pigs have a high requirement for vitamin C. Although proprietary packaged food will contain vitamin C, this may deteriorate during storage. Give fresh sources of vitamin C as described on page 12, or add a vitamin supplement.

• Some specific vitamins are particularly useful to boost the immune system, especially at times of stress.

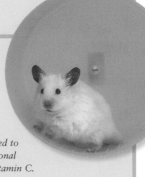

Hamsters need to be fed additional sources of vitamin C.

• For most pets, a general multivitamin and mineral supplement will support the immune system and be a useful addition to an average diet. If you are quite certain your pet is getting a fully balanced, organic, natural diet, this may not be vital, but few of us can be sure that our pets' diets are that perfect all year round.

VITAMINS

Because the vitamin and mineral requirements of pets varies from species to species, it is logical to obtain your supplement from your vet or a pet shop, where you can buy supplements specifically designed for different pets.

VITAMIN C
• Vitamin C is an antioxidant, which helps protect the body against disease. It promotes iron absorption, maintains healthy skin and fur, and is important in the production of antistress hormones.
• Vitamin C is not stored in the body, and is therefore almost impossible to overdose. However, very high doses occasionally cause diarrhea.
• There is no "ideal" protective dose of vitamin C, but an average daily supplement recommended is 100 mg per 11 lb (5 kg) bodyweight.

VITAMIN E
• Vitamin E is also an antioxidant, helping to fight infection and disease, and to neutralize the effects of pollutants. Best given in its natural form – look for the term "d-alpha-tocopherol" on the label. A suitable daily dose is 25 iu (international units) per 11 lb (5 kg) bodyweight.

VITAMIN B-COMPLEX
• Vitamin B-complex – the B vitamins as a group are important in keeping enzymes and metabolic pathways of the body working efficiently.
• Vitamin B-complex helps to repair body tissues, improves digestion, and keeps pets alert and energetic.
• Often given in the form of Brewers' yeast, a natural supplement very rich in B vitamins.
• Add ½tsp per 11 lb (5 kg) bodyweight to the food each day.
Other vitamins may be needed in specific situations. For instance, a combination of vitamins A, B, C, and E, with the mineral selenium, is recommended for severe immune system damage.

OTHER IMMUNE SYSTEM SUPPLEMENTS

Royal jelly is a substance secreted by worker bees to feed the larvae of the queen bee. It is rich in nutrients and enhances the functioning of the immune system. It improves the appetite when pets are not eating well, and increases energy in dull, depressed pets. Given regularly, it not only boosts the immune system but improves skin and coat condition. Give 1¾ oz (50g) fresh (not freeze-dried) royal jelly per 11 lb (5 kg) bodyweight daily.

Chlorella is a green alga containing nutrients. It can improve healing, help neutralize toxins, and boost the immune system. Give 1 g per 11 lb (5 kg) bodyweight daily.

Kelp is a powder produced from seaweed and is rich in vitamins and minerals. It aids red blood cell production, and maintains efficient functioning of many hormones and enzymes. Give 1 teaspoon per 11 lb (5 kg) bodyweight daily.

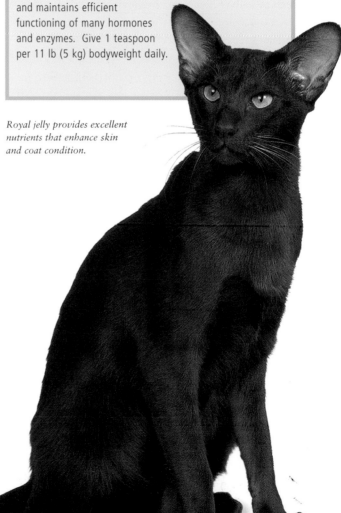

Royal jelly provides excellent nutrients that enhance skin and coat condition.

Home Environment

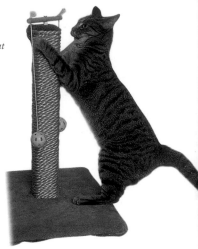

Indoor cats will benefit from toys and accessories that stimulate them.

Correct housing and proper exercise are important for all pets. It is essential to clean all cages, baskets, or other housing areas safely and regularly.

DOGS

Most dogs live indoors these days, but this is a fairly recent innovation. A few decades ago, most dogs lived in outdoor kennels – and on the whole were probably healthier for it. They had good ventilation, no exposure to central heating, air-conditioning, or cigarette smoke. However, since most of us prefer to have our dogs in the home with us, remember the following points:

• Ensure your dog has a suitable sleeping area, free of drafts, but not right next to a heating boiler that could produce fumes.

• If your dog has a sensitive skin, wash bedding in a non-biological detergent.

• Use humidifiers if the air is very dry as a result of central heating or air-conditioning.

• However warm and cosy the home is, dogs need exercise. Even for small dogs, a regular walk is essential. For some breeds, such as Border Collies, a lot of exercise is required to keep them physically and mentally healthy.

• Regularity is the keyword – not just a long walk at the weekend, but some exercise each day.

Dogs should have a draft-free sleeping area, away from direct heat. Natural bedding material is a healthier and more comfortable option.

CATS

Ideally, cats should be kept in a covered, secure run in a garden or yard. In practice, many cats are brought up indoors. They can on the whole cope well with this and can have a full, happy life. But they must be provided with sufficient stimulation. Some cats do need to explore the outside world and become restless and unhappy indoors. Cats that have been used to going outside may not adapt to an indoor life. Remember that cats are instinctive hunters, and like to lie in wait for their prey. Even indoors, they like to have hiding places to stay in and also to retreat to when anxious.

They are instinctively clean but sometimes shy animals. If you have to keep your cat inside for any reason unexpectedly, provide a litter tray in a quiet spot out of usual thoroughfares. There are cats which will go for a walk with a harness and lead – this is a good idea where or when they cannot roam freely.

CAGE BIRDS

No cage is ever really large enough – all pet birds are fitter and healthier in an aviary. But if it has to be a cage, choose the largest possible and keep it well above ground level. Install perches of different diameters – natural twigs and branches are best – and avoid sudden changes in temperature in the room. Try and let the bird out of the cage to fly sometimes, but make sure all doors and windows are closed so it cannot escape from the room.

FERRETS

Ferrets need strong cages with one square yard (about one square meter) or more of surface area for a pair of ferrets. Use hay or straw for bedding. Ferrets can cope with cold temperatures (though not freezing), but are susceptible to heat, so never have a cage in the direct sun. Access to exercise areas must be available. If trained from young, ferrets will use litter boxes and can live indoors.

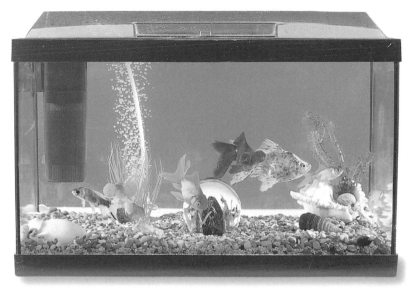

RABBITS, RODENTS, AND GUINEA PIGS

These pets are usually kept in cages or hutches. These must be spacious and kept in a safe place, out of reach from young children, and away from extremes of heat and cold.

• Chinchillas need a lot of space. They also need daily dust baths. Avoid high temperatures.

• Gerbils need solid-floored cages, and deep bedding for burrowing. Glass aquaria are ideal. Avoid metal bars, which cause sores to the nose.

• Guinea pigs can cope with a range of temperatures, but are better kept indoors in the winter. A mobile run that can be moved around a lawn is ideal.

• Rabbits should never be kept all their lives in a small hutch. They need a large run to which they have access regularly. Preferably they should live indoors – they can be house-trained – with access to an outdoor run.

• Rats and mice will chew through wood and plaster, so metal or glass cages are preferable. Like all rodents, they do need plenty of space for exercise.

• Hamsters also need space and a strong cage. Bedding is particularly important. Avoid cotton wool, which can cause constipation, and any material with strands that can tangle around legs.

Purchase a spacious, filtered tank for your fish.

FISH

Fish need large tanks, or ponds – never bowls. Water filtration systems to keep the water clean and pure are essential, and a regular water change is important. The best method is to change some of the water every week.

TORTOISES AND TERRAPINS

Tortoises need safe enclosures, with a shelter available and somewhere safe, dry, and frost-free to hibernate.

Terrapins require water, with a filtration system, and controlled water-heating. They also need a dry area out of the water available, preferably under an infrared lamp.

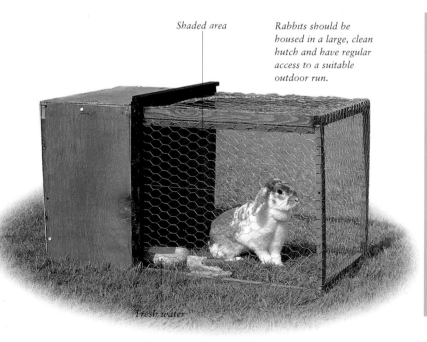

Shaded area

Rabbits should be housed in a large, clean hutch and have regular access to a suitable outdoor run.

Fresh water

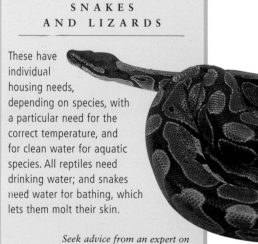

SNAKES AND LIZARDS

These have individual housing needs, depending on species, with a particular need for the correct temperature, and for clean water for aquatic species. All reptiles need drinking water; and snakes need water for bathing, which lets them molt their skin.

Seek advice from an expert on the correct type of housing for your species of reptile.

Pollutants and Negative Energies

Today, we are bombarded by a ceaseless flow of chemical pollutants, fertilizers, and electromagnetic radiation. At the same time, one of the main growth areas in disease is in immune system problems. Many illnesses are now recognized as being caused by a breakdown or malfunction of the immune system. Although it is sometimes difficult to prove a connection, there are many proven links, and much circumstantial evidence, that pollutants and background electromagnetic radiation are a big factor in the onset of immune system disease.

Remedies and supplements to help prevent, and treat, immune system disease are discussed on pages 156-161. This particular chapter explains what some of the trigger factors may be, and gives ways to prevent them affecting your pet.

Pollutants can be ingested by grooming.

ENVIRONMENTAL POLLUTION

Even the countryside is not the safe haven it used to be and there are many potentially damaging hazards to be avoided. Do not walk dogs over fields where fertilizer or lime has recently been laid, or spraying recently been carried out.

Factory chemicals and traffic fumes are a risk. Reduce the number of walks when air quality is poor. In icy weather, avoid walking dogs where thare has been recent salt treatment – this can cause damage to the feet.

Geopathic stress is another reaction to radiation. In some cases, chronic illness in pets (or humans) can be traced to imbalances in the background electromagnetic radiation of the earth below the home. Devices to neutralize this "geopathic stress" are available.

OUTDOORS

The damage to the ozone layer means that the sun's rays are more likely to cause sunburn, or heat stroke, in a shorter time than used to be the case.

• White cats are prone to cancer of the ear flap as a result of exposure to the sun.

LEFT *A clean and unpolluted environment will make a significant difference to the health of your dog.*

BELOW *Unless you are sure it is unpolluted, do not let dogs drink from ponds and lakes.*

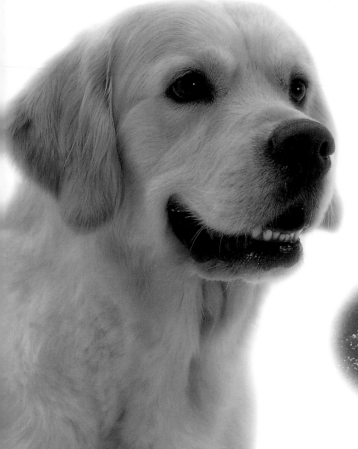

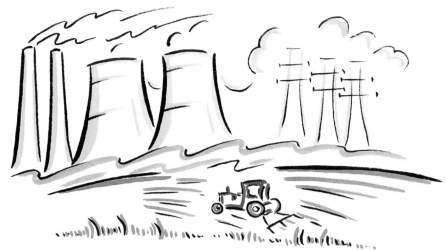

Do not walk dogs near nuclear power stations or other sources of radiation such as electricity pylons and cables.

• Some breeds of dogs (especially Border Collies) are prone to a serious inflammation of the nose, partly as a reaction to the sun.

• Dogs and cats do not sweat, so run more of a risk of heat-stroke than humans.

• Pets left in cars, even for short periods, on warm days, can quickly become heat exhausted.

So, welcome though sunshine is, be aware of its possible effects on your pet.

• Use sunblock cream on unprotected skin that may be affected by the sun.

• All small pets with outdoor runs must have a shaded shelter available. Rabbits, guinea pigs, and tortoises are susceptible to flies in hot weather. Flies lay eggs on moist areas, usually the anus, and maggots may develop as a result. Check small pets frequently in hot weather for signs of fly eggs or maggots.

• Overweight pets, or those with heart or respiratory problems, are particularly at risk.

INDOORS

If not treated with care, your own home is not necessarily a safer place to be than outdoors.

• Avoid using chemical sprays – hairsprays, fly sprays, and air fresheners.

• Carpet-freshening powders can often cause skin irritation in pets even after vacuuming it out of the carpet.

• Cage birds are easily poisoned by the fumes from non-stick cooking utensils – keep them well away from cooking areas and ensure adequate ventilation.

• The dry air caused by central heating can predispose to respiratory and skin problems. Use humidifiers if the air is very dry. However, chinchillas need a low humidity to keep skin and fur in good condition, and parrots that cough may be mimicking their owners, rather than suffering from a respiratory condition.

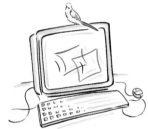

Computers and televisions create electromagnetic radiation, which can be harmful.

• Fish are especially susceptible to chemicals from sprays that settle on their water – cover fish tanks if any chemicals are being used in or near their tank.

• Good ventilation is always essential, but more so if anyone in the home smokes.

• Ionizers, which freshen the air, are a good investment, if air quality is a problem.

• Avoid overcrowding pets, especially fish and any pets kept in numbers in cages, such as gerbils.

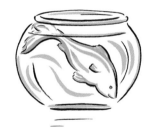

Fish are susceptible to any chemical sprays that settle on the surface of their water. A covered aquarium or tank is a better container for them.

• Ferrets are prone to zinc poisoning from licking cage bars or galvanized feeding dishes.

• Feeding utensils for all pets should be stainless steel or ceramic; plastic and other materials can leach chemicals into food or water.

• Electromagnetic radiation from computers and televisions can be harmful. Keep small pets cages well away from these and other items of electrical equipment. Quartz crystals placed on computers and televisions will absorb some of this negative radiation.

MENTAL WELL-BEING

As well as having good food and good housing, pets need mental stimulation, companionship, and freedom from stress.

DOGS

• Dogs thrive on the close bond between themselves and their human carers. But just walking the dog is not enough – dogs need to play, chase, and to be trained. Most dogs want to please. Training and obedience classes don't sound like fun to us, but most dogs enjoy it and are stimulated mentally by the continuing process of obedience training.

• If a dog has to be left alone in the home, provide toys that stimulate the senses.

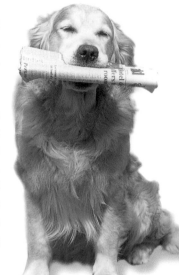

• Some breeds need much more mental stimulation than others – Border Collies, for instance.

• Regular grooming of dogs is an important part of the time you spend with them. It not only helps keep skin in good condition and the coat glossy, but also promotes a sense of well-being in the dog.

• Dogs that enjoy meeting and playing with other dogs should be given the opportunity to do so. Some dogs are very sociable, some are only happy in human company. Respect their needs.

Most dogs want to please and are mentally stimulated by training and obedience classes and interaction with their owners.

Kittens enjoy playing with toys and benefit from the stimulation.

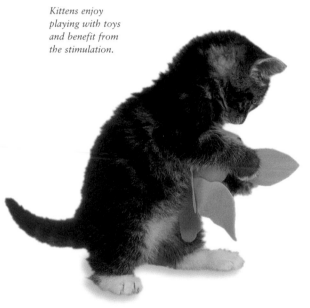

CATS

• Cats may seem to be more independent and less playful than dogs, but do need mental stimulation too. They usually enjoy play that mimics their natural hunting activities – chasing or throwing toy "prey" around.

• Cats are not as naturally sociable as dogs and become stressed in many situations. Make sure they have an area they can retreat into when stressed, and use stress-relieving remedies if any disruption in their lives occurs.

RODENTS AND SMALL ANIMALS

• Chinchillas are acrobatic, energetic creatures, and need lots of space to indulge in physical activity. They are not stressed by handling. (But if handled roughly, patches of fur will come off in your hand – this is called furslip.)

• Gerbils are burrowing animals and need to be able to do this for their mental well-being. There must be sufficient depth and type of material in their cage.

• Gerbils live in groups happily, but if one is removed and then re-introduced later, they may fight. Provide hiding places in the cage for any subordinate individuals.

• Hamsters are solitary animals and usually need to be kept on their own. They can be aggressive toward each other, so do not stress them by trying to keep them together.

• Hamsters scent-mark their environment. Excessive cleaning of their cage will disturb and upset them.

• Guinea pigs are sociable pets and can be kept in groups. They are one of the more interactive of the small pets, and if handled regularly, will enjoy human attention.

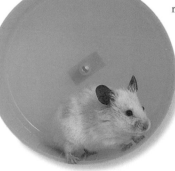

Hamsters are solitary animals that are best kept in separate cages.

• Rabbits make very good indoor pets, responding to space and mental stimulation and often becoming depressed or aggressive if deprived of space and companionship.

• Rats and mice are sociable beings, and rats particularly enjoy human company and interaction. They rarely bite if they are used to being handled.

• Ferrets also respond to regular handling, and rarely bite when used to human contact.

• All small pets need an environment that is interesting and provides mental stimulation, and where changes are made regularly to prevent boredom. Change toys frequently – but avoid any change that may be stressful, such as moving the place where the pet normally sleeps.

• Cage birds need variety – have a rota of toys to provide stimulation. Avoid rubber toys and be careful of chains with links that could get caught in the bird's leg band. A change of scenery often livens up a depressed bird – move the cage to a different room, or nearer a window. Make sure this doesn't mean a sudden change in temperature, and that it is not into an area where cooking is done. There is a risk of poisoning from fumes when heating non-stick utensils.

Rats enjoy human company and rarely bite if they are used to being handled.

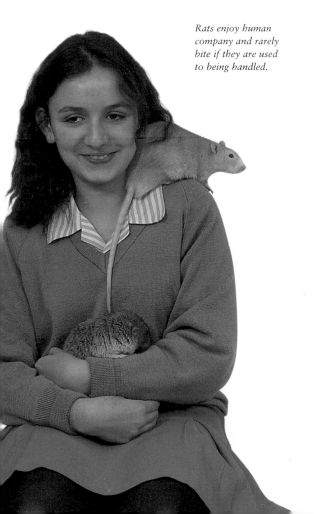

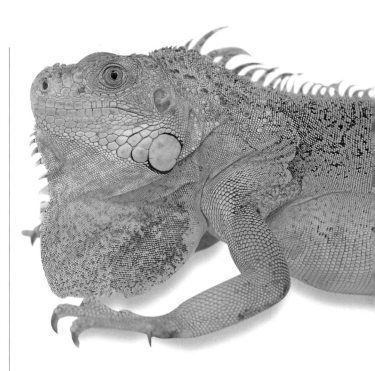

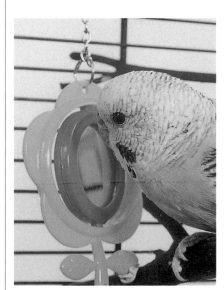

ABOVE *To keep your reptile mentally healthy, ensure that it has the right environment for its particular needs.*

LEFT *Caged birds respond well to a rotation of stimulating toys, such as mirrors.*

REPTILES

• Reptiles have differing needs. Some are burrowing, some need to climb, some are mainly aquatic. Find out the usual habitat of your tortoise, terrapin, snake, or lizard and provide an environment as close to it as possible. Cold blooded animals need stimulation too.

FISH

• Fish need space – overcrowding is the main risk to mental well-being. They also need some water furniture to make their lives more interesting.

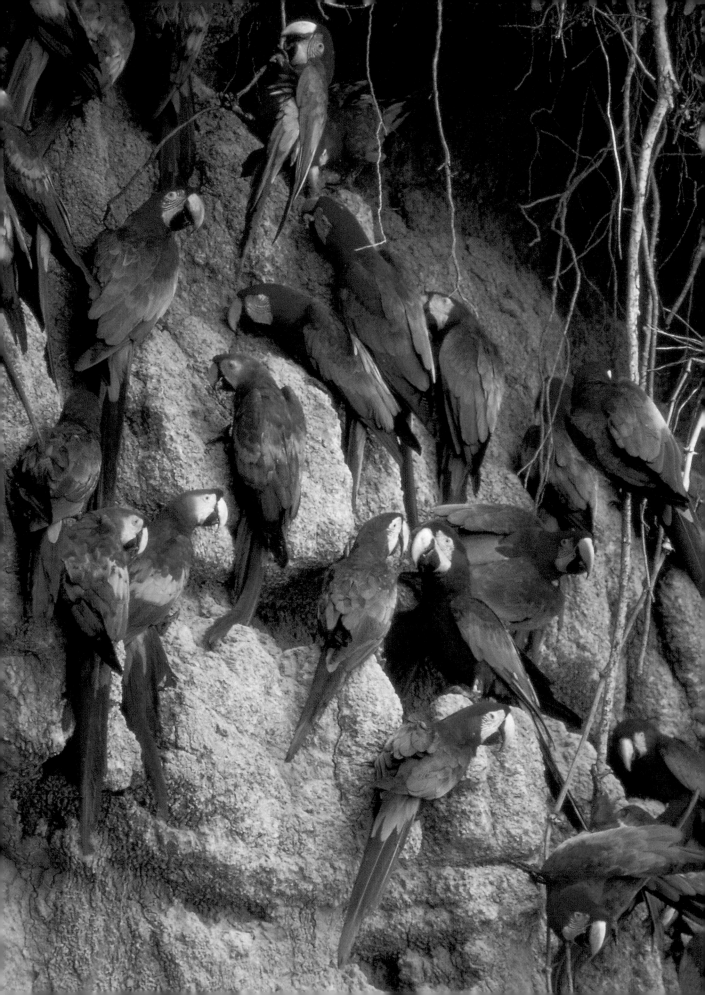

Part II

Natural Therapies

Natural therapies are not a replacement for appropriate veterinary treatment when needed. Never be tempted to avoid a visit to the veterinarian solely by using this book. But the therapies that follow can be used in addition to any necessary veterinary treatment, to speed up the healing process, and for minor problems where veterinary treatment would not be necessary. The most important point to remember is – if in doubt, always consult your veterinarian. Don't risk your pet's health because you want to save time or money by delaying veterinary attention, or because you "prefer" natural medicines.

That said, it is equally important to consider using natural medicine where possible and appropriate. There are many drawbacks to conventional medicine. Drugs are powerful – and they may have side-effects.

In addition, conventional drugs tend to be suppressive. They often inhibit the immune system at the same time as attacking the inflammation or the infection. This means other diseases can get a hold, and certain organs, such as the liver or kidneys, may be damaged by the drug.

HEALING NATURALLY

By comparison, natural remedies are invariably gentle in their action, when administered correctly. Most are holistic, acting on the whole body rather than simply on part of it. They stimulate the body to heal itself, rather than treating the body as a battleground on which the drug is at war with the condition.

If conventional drugs are being administered, none of the therapies listed here will have an adverse effect on the action of the drug being used. However, it is advisable to inform your veterinarian of any remedy you are adding to the prescribed treatment. Some conventional drugs do reduce the effectiveness of natural medicines. For example, steroids suppress the beneficial effect of some remedies, particularly homeopathic medicines. Most natural therapies are

Animals in the wild instinctively select roots and vegetation to cure ailments.

compatible with each other, but there are some exceptions. Strongly scented essential oils and herbs will reduce the efficacy of homeopathic remedies.

HEALING SAFELY

Natural therapies have many advantages – they are extremely effective, safe and free from side-effects, easily available in pet shops, pharmacies, or health food stores, and their production is not dependant on animal-tested substances, nor does it pollute the earth.

However, natural remedies are safe and free from side-effects only when used properly. Herbs, if given in overdose, can be toxic. Essential oils are poisonous if swallowed in more than very small amounts. A homeopathic remedy given for too long may cause an aggravation of symptoms. Follow the advice given in this guide and your pet will be safe – but don't assume all remedies are automatically safe, and always administer them according to the directions.

There is a tremendous range of natural remedies and therapies to help a sick pet. Some therapies, such as acupuncture, should be administered only by a trained practitioner, but most, ranging from aromatherapy to homeopathy, may be used following the guidelines in this book.

Animals in the wild naturally select the herbs, roots, berries, and grasses to cure their ailments. Our domestic pets don't have access to these natural medicines, but now we can provide them. We also have access to other natural therapies – manipulative treatment such as osteopathy and chiropractic; energy medicines such as crystal therapy and magnet therapy.

Our pets deserve the benefits that safe, effective natural therapies can give them when they are ill. People are turning more and more to natural medicines for themselves. We shouldn't allow our pets to be left out!

Using natural therapies means your pet will recover more quickly, but without the danger of side-effects that can arise using conventional medicine only. From the smallest fish to the largest St Bernard dog, there is always a natural therapy to use.

Acupuncture and Acupressure

The word acupuncture combines the Latin *acu*, "with a needle" and the word "puncture." The process of acupuncture involves inserting fine needles into specific points on the body. These points are along channels known as meridians, which are essentially energy flows through the body. By inserting needles into these energy channels, the flow of energy can be increased, decreased, or balanced, in order to stimulate healing.

Acupuncture has been used for thousands of years and its benefits are well known. Although it can be used to treat virtually any illness or disease, it is best known for its effectiveness in relieving pain and in treating disorders of muscles, bones, joints, and nerves.

• Arthritis, back problems, muscle cramps, and injured nerves respond particularly well to acupuncture.

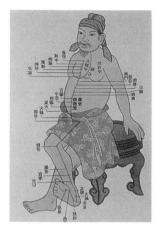

Acupuncture points were first recognized in Chinese medicine.

• Acupuncture is suitable for most species.
• Needles are made of stainless steel or copper, and can be anything from ½ inch (12mm) to 1 inch (25mm) in length.
• Needles are disposable and never used more than once.
• Needles are left in place for 5–20 minutes, depending on the problem and patient being treated.
• Because the needles are so fine, bleeding from a needle puncture is extremely rare.
• Sometimes improvement can take a little while to be seen. It is usually worthwhile to have three sessions of acupuncture before assessing results.
• Occasionally symptoms become worse before getting better, again be patient
• Smaller pets, and obviously pets such as fish and tortoises, are not suitable candidates for acupuncture.

THE TWELVE MERIDIANS

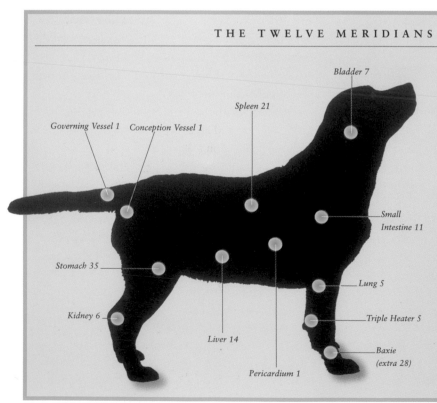

Bladder 7

Spleen 21

Governing Vessel 1 *Conception Vessel 1*

Small Intestine 11

Stomach 35

Lung 5

Kidney 6

Triple Heater 5

Liver 14

Baxie (extra 28)

Pericardium 1

• There are twelve pairs of meridians – bladder, lung, liver, gall-bladder, pericardium, small intestine, large intestine, heart, kidney, stomach, spleen, triple heater – and two single meridians – conception vessel and governing vessel.

• The names of the meridians are no clue to their actual use in acupuncture. For instance, the bladder meridian has many points used to treat arthritis and other joint problems. Some examples of meridian points are labeled opposite.

• The decision on which points to use is made by reference to a complex series of rules taken from Traditional Chinese Medicine – it takes years of practice to master.

• Dogs and rabbits accept acupuncture surprisingly well.

• Only a veterinarian trained in acupuncture should be permitted to carry out acupuncture on animals. Do not try acupuncture yourself!

Apart from straightforward needling, there are other methods of stimulating the points:

• Electro-acupuncture involves applying a small electric current via an electrode attached to the needle, so amplifying the stimulating effect.

• Laser acupuncture is the use of a laser beam at the acupunture point, rather than a needle. This is not invasive, but involves the use of specialized equipment, which can mean an expensive procedure.

• Aquapuncture involves injecting a fluid into the acupuncture point. Usually either vitamin B12 or herbal extracts are injected. These potentiate the effect of the acupuncture. It is often useful for pets, for it is an "instant" treatment, meaning that the patient does not have to stay still while needles are left in place.

• Acupressure is the technique of applying pressure at the various acupuncture points, rather than stimulating with a needle, laser, or Moxa. Pressure is applied with a finger or the thumb. It is the only version of acupuncture that is safe for use at home.

• Rubbing or pressing any spot that hurts is a natural, unconscious form of acupressure.

The exact mechanism of action of acupuncture and its variants is not fully understood. It has been proven that certain acupuncture points, when stimulated, cause the release of endorphins, the body's natural painkillers.

There is a difference in the electrical potential of the skin over an acupuncture point, which can be measured. It is therefore likely that the energy flow disturbed by this ancient Chinese practice is something akin to an electric current flowing around the body and controlling body processes, just as electricity "controls" electrical equipment. Acupuncture lets this energy flow be balanced,

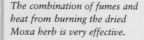

MOXIBUSTION

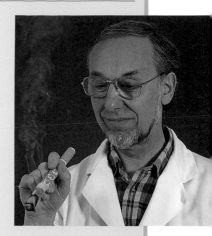

• Moxibustion is the practice of burning the dried herb Moxa, and applying this to the needle. The heat that then travels down the needle, as well as the fumes of the smoldering Moxa, enhances the healing effect. Moxa can also be applied to the skin directly.

The combination of fumes and heat from burning the dried Moxa herb is very effective.

smooth, and with maximum current, so stimulating healing, relieving pain, and repairing damage in the whole body.

Not only do most animal patients accept acupuncture well, but in many cases the needling is calming and invokes a sense of well-being, especially in pets that are in pain. Some patients come to look forward to their sessions!

For advice and availability of acupuncture therapy, consult your local veterinary practice or the national Veterinary Acupuncture Association. Many veterinarians who specialize in acupunture have an IVAS Certificate, denoting a high standard of competence.

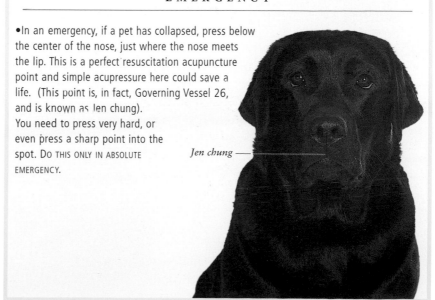

EMERGENCY

•In an emergency, if a pet has collapsed, press below the center of the nose, just where the nose meets the lip. This is a perfect resuscitation acupuncture point and simple acupressure here could save a life. (This point is, in fact, Governing Vessel 26, and is known as Jen chung).
You need to press very hard, or even press a sharp point into the spot. DO THIS ONLY IN ABSOLUTE EMERGENCY.

Jen chung

Light, Color, and Magnetic Therapy

LIGHT THERAPY

This is more accurately termed "low-energy photon therapy," and is a form of laser treatment. The lasers emit either visible (orange-red) or invisible laser light. Their focused light has a healing effect on damaged tissue.

• Light therapy can be used to stimulate acupuncture points. This is non-invasive and painless and therefore useful for nervous or highly-strung patients.

• The low-energy lasers used in light therapy will not cause a heat increase in the animal.

• All lasers should be kept away from the eyes.

• Laser treatment should only be carried out by a skilled, trained practitioner.

• Light therapy is anti-inflammatory and reduces edema. It works by increasing blood and lymphatic flow through the affected tissue, thereby removing toxins and excess fluid.

• Light treatment stimulates regeneration of damaged nerves and is particularly useful for nerve injuries following accidents and injuries. Similarly, damaged muscles and tendons heal and regenerate in response to light therapy.

• Laser therapy is especially effective in treating ulcers, non-healing wounds and burns, as well as scar tissue.

• Laser light machines are now, in most cases, produced in small, portable forms, including a pen laser.

• Light therapy is suitable for all pets, except fish.

• A low-output, battery-operated, pocket-sized laser pen is safe for home use for first aid treatment – wounds, scratches, inflamed ears – but not as a replacement for veterinary treatment.

Advice in the use of a laser therapy must be obtained from a skilled practitioner before use.

COLOR THERAPY

Colored, non-laser light or even color in the form of colored fabrics can be used as a healing agent. Each color of the spectrum has its own individual effect

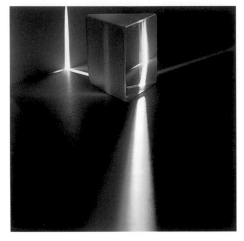

The full spectrum of color can be used to heal.

on physical and mental well-being, and has its own energy, which interacts with that of the patient in a positive way.

• Color can be applied in the form of a light shone onto the patient, or simply by letting the pet lie or sleep on a blanket or rug of the required color.

• The color red increases energy and enhances the life force.

• Blue is a calming, healing color. It is beneficial for diseases such as epilepsy and acute diarrhea.

• Green is a balancing color and assists heart disease and trauma.

• Orange is effective for anemia and for fears and phobias.

• Yellow is used in the treatment of eczema and cataracts.

• Indigo is the color for eye and ear disease.

• Violet is a relaxing color and treats kidney problems and sinusitis.

• Metallic gold is good for infections and acute fevers.

• Metallic silver helps heal fractures and other bone injuries.

• A person specializing in color therapy is called a chromopractitioner, and such a specialist should be consulted when actual light sources are used.

• Color therapy is applicable to all pets – even fish can benefit from colored light for short periods of time.

Color therapy is suitable for all animals.

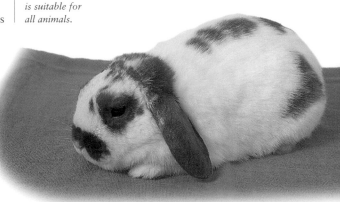

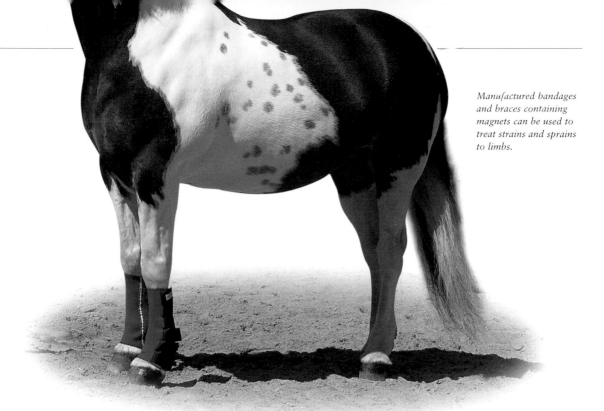

Manufactured bandages and braces containing magnets can be used to treat strains and sprains to limbs.

MAGNETIC THERAPY

Blood contains hemoglobin, which in turn contains iron. It is therefore not surprising that magnets have a major effect on the body, and on circulation in particular. Magnetism has been used for centuries as a cure for a variety of disorders. Two major forms of magnetic therapies are in use – static magnets and pulsed electromagnetic field magnets (PEMF). In each case, the magnet is placed on or near the area to be treated. Magnetic lines of force emanate from the magnet and infiltrate the damaged area to promote healing and aid recovery.

• Magnetic therapy works by improving the circulation to the affected areas, removing toxins and excess fluid.

• Static magnets are permanently magnetized and do not need to be replaced. They can be left in place for hours or days – or even permanently, in the case of ongoing conditions such as arthritis.

• Collars containing magnets, which pets such as dogs and cats can wear continuously, are now available. They are ideal for the older animal with chronic arthritis or other long-term health problems.

• PEMF magnets are more powerful but need an electrical supply; battery-powered models are now in use. Sessions usually last 30 minutes to 1 hour, and the patient obviously needs to stay still during the treatment.

• Magnetic therapy is most beneficial for musculoskeletal problems – hip dysplasia in dogs; spinal conditions such as spondylosis in most pets; arthritis, sprains, and strains in most species.

• Apart from collars, magnets can be sewn into harnesses for larger pets to wear, and wraps containing magnets which can be wrapped around damaged limbs or the whole body are available from specialist manufacturers.

• PEMF magnets should preferably be used by physio-therapists, or others skilled in the use of these devices.

• Magnetic therapy should not be used on fresh wounds or injuries – start only after the first two days of healing. The increase in blood supply to a fresh wound or injury may initially cause too much swelling or bleeding.

• Do not use magnet therapy on pregnant pets – or any animals with a pacemaker or other artificial heart device.

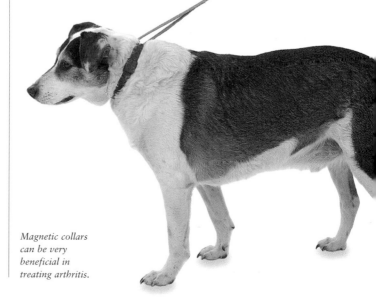

Magnetic collars can be very beneficial in treating arthritis.

Aromatherapy

Aromatherapy is the use of volatile essential oils from plants in the treatment of disease. The oils are obtained by distillation, by pressing, or by extraction using solvents. Because a large volume of plant material is needed to produce a small amount of oil, they are often expensive to manufacture and therefore buy.

OILS

Oils are obtained from flowers, buds, fruits, leaves, and other parts of the plant. Whenever possible, they should be obtained from organically grown plants. Organic oils are of better quality, and are also free from herbicides and pesticides, which could survive the extraction process. Synthetic essential oils are also available. These are cheaper, pure, and free from pesticides – but are simply not as effective as organic essentials oils.

Each oil has its own individual properties that address different mental, emotional, and physical conditions. However, as a general guide, all oils are antiseptic and detoxifying, and all help strengthen the immune system and equalize metabolism. The precise method of action on the body is unknown, but as with all natural therapies, their effectiveness seems to hinge on the interaction of the energy in the remedy with the energy in the patient. This interaction creates a healing effect.

There are two main ways of administering essential oils – massage and diffusion. Although oils may be taken by mouth, this is not normally recommended because even small amounts can be toxic.

MASSAGE

Massage is not always feasible for pets with thick fur, feathers, or scales. However, for dogs and cats it is usually an enjoyable method. To prepare for massage, add a drop of each oil to be used to ½ teaspoon of an inert carrier oil (wheatgerm, grapeseed, sweet almond, or sunflower). This carrier dilutes the oil making it safer and letting it be absorbed more easily through the skin. Choose a hairless, or thinly coated, area of skin. Massage a few drops of the diluted mixture into the area for three to four minutes. Repeat this process twice daily for four days, less if the symptoms resolve. Clean

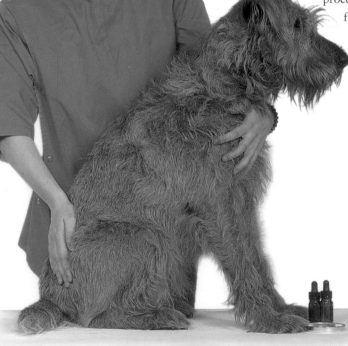

Massage is an effective and enjoyable method of administering aromatherapy.

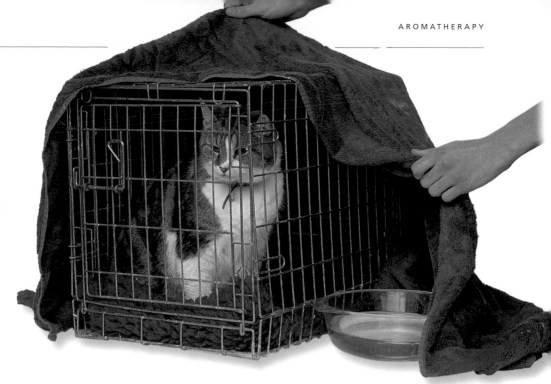

RIGHT *Essential oils can be effectively administered using a diffuser to vaporize the oil for short periods of time.*

LEFT *Pure essential oils are more effective that synthetic alternatives. Always store them away from direct sulight.*

the skin well after massage to avoid the pet licking and swallowing oils. Never apply neat essentials oils directly onto the skin. Because there has been little use of essential oils in animals apart from dogs and cats, and the effect on other smaller mammals and birds is not fully understood, it is not recommended to massage oils into other pets.

DIFFUSION

Diffusion is probably the ideal way of administering oils. A diffuser can be as simple as a candle heating a small bowl of the diluted oil. Alternatively, an electric diffuser can be used this heats the oil without the danger of a naked flame. An even simpler method is to soak some cotton wool with diluted oil and place it (out of the pet's reach) in the room. Dogs and cats should not be exposed to the oil vapor for long periods – 15–20 minutes a day is sufficient and other smaller pets should be exposed to diffused oils for only very short periods – a minute or two at a time, repeated over a course, until healing is complete.

• When using homeopathy, the following essential oils will reduce the effectiveness of the remedies – black pepper, camphor, eucalyptus, peppermint.

• Oils that can cause an adverse reaction if used before exposure to sunlight are angelica root, bergamot, lime, bitter orange, lemon, grapefruit, sweet orange, and tangerine.

• If a pet accidentally swallows any oil, get veterinary attention as soon as possible and make a note of which oil or oils have been swallowed.

• Cats have a sensitivity to phenols, naturally occurring chemicals found in some plants. Oils containing phenols are cinnamon leaf, sweet fennel, parsley seed, West Indian bay, aniseed, and clove.

ADVERSE REACTIONS

If any pet appears to have an adverse reaction to essential oils, stop using them immediately. Oils most likely to cause skin irritation are benzoin, lemon eucalyptus, melissa, tagetes, valerian, and yarrow. Cats sometimes react to tea tree oil. DO NOT USE ESSENTIAL OILS ON PREGNANT ANIMALS. Animals that are epileptic can safely be given all essential oils except fennel, hyssop, rosemary, and Spanish sage.

Eucalyptus

Angelica

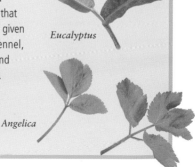

A lampshade collar prevents cats from licking their fur.

INDIVIDUAL OILS – THEIR USES AND PROPERTIES

ANGELICA ROOT
Poor skin condition, long-standing eczema, bronchitis, coughs, anemia, flatulence.
A good calming agent for stress and anxiety. Restorative and revitalizing for pets with low energy levels.
DO NOT USE ON DIABETIC PETS.

ANISEED
Muscle damage, arthritis, poor circulation, bronchitis, coughs, colitis, colic, and flatulence.
A warming, soothing, comforting oil. Occasionally causes skin reactions. Use in very small amounts and check carefully for any skin irritation if used for massage.

BASIL, SWEET/FRENCH
Good insect repellent, immune system booster, arthritis, muscular cramps, sinusitis.
An uplifting remedy for dull, depressed pets.
Combine with citronella and virginia cedarwood to produce a good repellent for biting flies in summer.

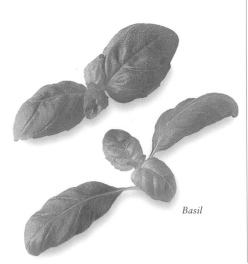

Basil

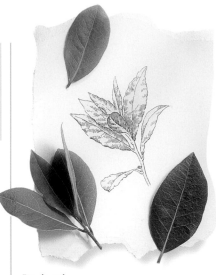

Bay laurel

BAY, WEST INDIAN
Good stimulant for pets with poor skin condition. Heals scurfy and scaling skin, promotes hair growth, reduces seborrhea. Also useful for sprains and strains.
USE IN VERY SMALL AMOUNTS; OCCASIONAL SKIN REACTIONS HAVE OCCURRED.

BENZOIN
Good respiratory remedy, for asthma, bronchitis, influenza, and coughs.
A warming, stimulating oil. Helps relieve stress and tension.
USE BY DIFFUSION ONLY – CAN CAUSE SKIN IRRITATION.

BERGAMOT
Excellent mouth and throat remedy – good for bad breath, sore gums, sore throat, and tonsillitis. A good immune system booster; also treats cystitis.
CAN SENSITIZE SKIN TO SUNLIGHT, SO AVOID USING FOR MASSAGE.

CAJEPUT
Greasy, oily skin. A good respiratory remedy – catarrh and sinusitis, recurrent sore throats, asthma. Also urinary infections.
OCCASIONAL CASE OF SKIN IRRITATION AFTER USE.

CAMPHOR, WHITE
Arthritis, sprains, and strains. Good for sudden onset of fevers and chills. Also for chronic eczema.

Brown and yellow camphor are toxic and should never be used.

CARDAMOM
Excellent digestive remedy, for loss of appetite, colic and colitis, vomiting, bad breath, gas in the bowels.
STRONG SMELL BUT NON-IRRITATING. USE FOR SHORT PERIODS ONLY.

CARROT SEED
Ideal oil for skin problems, eczema, rashes, greasy skin. Also good for hormonal imbalance in females. Combines well with cedarwood, geranium, and citrus oils.

CEDARWOOD, ATLAS
Another good skin remedy for flaking, greasy skin, for fungal infections, and for hair loss. Also for chest congestion and catarrh.
One of the tonic oils – revives and uplifts; good to relieve stress and tension.

CELERY SEED
Remedy for liver problems and digestive upsets, beneficial in glandular problems, increases milk flow in mammary glands. Useful when there is nerve inflammation (neuritis) and sudden shooting pains.

CAMOMILE, GERMAN (BLUE)
Useful remedy for nerve pains, toothache and teething pains, insect bites, wounds,

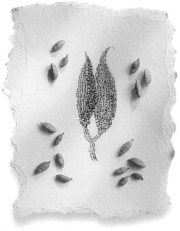

Cardamom seeds

muscular and joint pains, and pain from abscesses and burns.
A good stress-relieving remedy, helps pets sleep restfully.

CAMOMILE, ROMAN
Anti-inflammatory oil, for dermatitis, rashes, inflamed joints and muscles, and colitis.
VERY SAFE TO USE, BUT HAS OCCASIONALLY CAUSED SKIN REACTIONS.

CINNAMON LEAF
Good repellent against lice, mange mites, and fleas. Excellent for digestive problems, especially diarrhea and colitis. Helps stimulate contractions in pets giving birth.

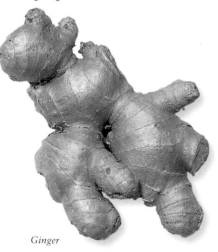

Ginger

CITRONELLA
Immune system booster, helps prevent and fight minor infections. Stimulates the nervous system, good for loss of energy. A good insect repellent when combined with virginian cedarwood.

CLOVE BUD
Helps heal ulcers, wounds, burns, cuts, sore gums, and bruises. Also for sprains and strains. A very strong oil – use very dilute, below 1%.

CORIANDER/CILANTRO
Circulatory remedy, helps remove excess fluids. Used for ascites (dropsy), swollen joints, poor circulation, and heart disease. Stimulatory oil for debilitated and weak pets

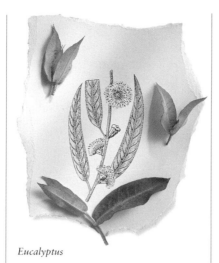

Eucalyptus

CYPRESS
Pyorrhea (gum infection), circulatory problems such as edema, and respiratory problems.
A good stress-relieving remedy for anxious pets.

DILL SEED
Mainly a digestive remedy for colitis and flatulence.
Also has the ability to increase milk flow from mammary glands.

ELEMI
"Rejuvenates" damaged skin, heals untreated cuts and wounds. Also for dry coughs and bronchitis.
A useful remedy for stressed and debilitated pets.

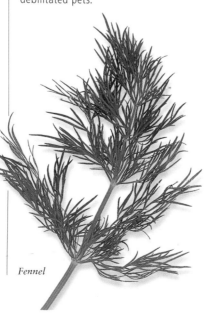

Fennel

EUCALYPTUS BLUE GUM
Especially for respiratory problems (asthma, coughs, sinusitis, throat infections); also for skin conditions.
USE VERY DILUTE – CAN IRRITATE THE SKIN.

FENNEL, SWEET
Digestive problems respond well (constipation, poor appetite, flatulence); also improves circulation.
DO NOT USE ON EPILEPTIC PETS.

FRANKINCENSE
Respiratory conditions (sore throats, bronchitis, asthma); also cystitis and other urinary problems.
Calms and slows breathing, good for anxious pets and pets with phobias.

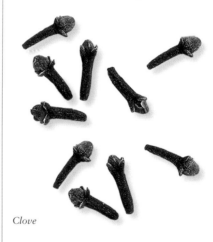

Clove

GALBANUM
Primarily for skin problems since it softens and heals damaged skin.
Good for abscesses, cuts, scars.
Useful as an insect repellent.

GERANIUM, ROSE
Helps hormonal imbalances, including adrenal gland problems. Also an invaluable skin remedy for ringworm, ulcers, wounds, and burns.
OCCASIONALLY CAUSES SKIN REACTIONS IN PETS WITH SENSITIVE SKIN.

GINGER
A stimulatory remedy, for the circulation, for muscular aches and pains, and for the digestion.
A useful remedy for pets suffering from travel sickness.

GRAPEFRUIT
A skin remedy, it tones skin and encourages hair growth. Also useful for older, overweight, stiff pets.
HAS A SHORT SHELF LIFE – QUICKLY OXIDIZES.

HYSSOP
Particularly useful for respiratory conditions (severe coughs, bronchitis, pharyngitis, tonsillitis).
DO NOT USE ON PETS WITH EPILEPSY.

JASMINE
Useful for uterine disorders; also for dry, sensitive, flaky skins, and for throat problems.
VERY OCCASIONALLY CAUSES ALLERGIC REACTIONS.

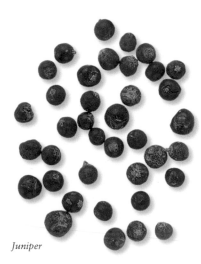

Juniper

JUNIPER
Excellent skin remedy (dermatitis, eczema, hair loss); also for the overweight pet with stiff joints.
AVOID USE OF JUNIPER ON PETS WITH KIDNEY DISEASE.

LAVENDER, TRUE
Probably the single most important skin remedy: treats ringworm, mange mites, sunburn, wounds, bruises, burns. Also for arthritis and respiratory disorders.
Can be used on the skin without need for dilution.

LEMON EUCALYPTUS
Fungal and yeast skin conditions, and for scabby, dry, crusty skins. Also for sore throats.
Another good insect repellent.

LEMONGRASS, WEST INDIAN
Treats fevers and infectious diseases. Also lice, scabies, and other parasitic skin diseases, poor muscular tone, gastroenteritis.
Good antiparasite remedy – fleas, lice, ticks.

LEMON
Astringent and refreshing; good for warts, broken nails, poor feather or scale condition, ulcers, and also nosebleeds. An immune system booster.
CAN CAUSE PHOTOSENSITIZATION (SKIN IRRITATION AFTER EXPOSURE TO SUN).

LIME
Asthma, bronchitis, catarrh, high blood pressure, nosebleeds, and congestion in the circulation.
PRESSED LIME OIL, BUT NOT DISTILLED LIME OIL, MAY CAUSE PHOTO-SENSITIZATION (SKIN IRRITATION AFTER EXPOSURE TO SUN).

MANDARIN
Fluid retention, obesity, scar tissue, and digestive problems.
A calming oil suitable for pets that are restless and don't sleep well.

MARJORAM, SWEET
Has many uses: arthritis, sprains and strains, general muscular stiffness and cramps, constipation and flatulence, coughs and flu, hormonal imbalances.
A good stress-relieving remedy.

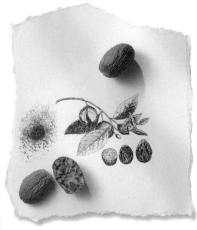

Nutmeg

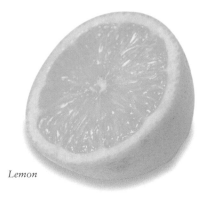

Lemon

MELISSA (LEMON BALM)
Allergies and insect stings, asthma, chronic coughs, colitis, vomiting, anxiety and nervousness, shock and trauma.
CAN IRRITATE SKIN SO USE IN LOW DILUTION (NO HIGHER THAN 1%).

MYRRH
Chronic respiratory symptom problems (persistent coughs, catarrh, sinusitis, nasal discharge). Boosts resistance to infection.
A mild, safe oil, suitable for repeated use.

NEROLI
Scar tissue, chronic diarrhea, colitis, flatulence. Nervous system problems (shock and fright, emotional traumas and depression).
An ideal stress-relieving remedy.

NUTMEG
Arthritis, muscular weakness, poor circulation, and constipation or sluggish digestion. Helps fight bacterial infection.
A tonic remedy for the heart, circulation, and the nerves.

ORANGE, SWEET
Mouth ulcers and gingivitis, fluid retention and obesity, constipation and sluggish digestion, tendency to respiratory infections, and dull, dry, or greasy skin.
Can cause photo-sensitivity, so caution when used during summer time.

PALMAROSA
Skin conditions (dermatitis, repeated skin infection, scar tissue, seborrhea). Loss of

appetite. General weakness and debility. Useful for pets suffering from repeated intestinal infections.

PARSLEY SEED
Antitoxin, so helps remove toxins from arthritic joints, relieves cystitis and other urinary problems, helps toxic digestive problems, colitis, and flatulence.
Helps promote a normal labor when pets are giving birth.

PATCHOULI
Primarily a skin remedy (wet eczema, open sores, ringworm and yeast infections, scurfy and scaly skin, cracked and fissured skin, wounds and bruises). Also a good remedy for nervousness and anxiety.

PEPPER, BLACK
Anemia, sprains, muscle stiffness, myositis. A good antiviral and antibacterial remedy. Loss of appetite. Colitis and diarrhea.
CAN BE IRRITANT – USE IN LOW CONCENTRATION (LESS THAN 1%).

PEPPERMINT
Abdominal cramps, colic, colitis, flatulence, vomiting. Bad breath. Fevers and sudden infections.
TOO POWERFUL TO BE USED AT THE SAME TIME AS HOMEOPATHIC REMEDIES.

PETITGRAIN, ORANGE
Greasy skin and coat, sleeplessness, stress remedy.
A good remedy to aid convalescence after major illnesses.

PINE NEEDLE, SCOTCH
Arthritis, stiff muscles, respiratory conditions (sinusitis, catarrh). Also parasitic skin conditions (mange, mites, lice).
CAN IRRITATE THE SKIN – USE IN LOW CONCENTRATIONS.

ROSE MAROC
Allergic respiratory conditions (asthma and hay fever-like symptoms). Liver disorders. Dry, flaky skin.
Soothing and calming.

ROSEMARY
Skin problems (eczema, mites, lice). Fluid retention. Severe coughs. Liver disease, jaundice. A good immune system booster at times of stress.
DO NOT USE ON EPILEPTIC PETS.

ROSEWOOD
Immune system stimulant. Fights fevers, sudden onset infections. Also a stress-relieving remedy.

SAGE, CLARY
Skin inflammation, dandruff and flaking, ulcers. Coughs and throat infections.

SAGE, SPANISH
Eczema, liver disease, jaundice. Coughs and laryngitis. Weakness and debility. A useful remedy for gingivitis and other gum problems.

SANDALWOOD
Dry, cracked skin, dry persistent coughs, diarrhea, cystitis.
Opens up airways and relieves respiratory congestion.

TAGETES
Thickened skin, calluses, fungal skin infections.
USE IN LOW CONCENTRATIONS – OCCASIONAL REPORTS OF SKIN IRRITATION.

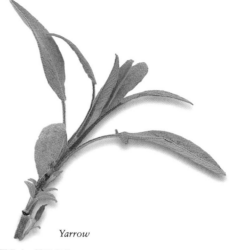
Yarrow

TEA TREE
Excellent natural antiseptic, antibacterial, antifungal, and antiviral agent. All infective problems, and most skin problems, respond to tea tree.
CAN BE USED UNDILUTED ON SKIN IN MOST CASES, BUT OCCASIONALLY CAUSES MILD IRRITATION.

THYME, WHITE
Skin conditions: abscesses, burns, cuts, eczema, insect stings. Arthritis, myositis, poor circulation.
USE IN LOW CONCENTRATION.

VALERIAN
Perfect remedy for sleeplessness, anxiety, nervousness, restlessness, and fears and phobias.
STRONG ODOR – USE FOR SHORT PERIODS ONLY.

VETIVERT
Wounds, cuts, bruises, sprains, stiffness, arthritis.
Known as the oil of tranquillity because of its ability to relieve stress, nervousness, and depression.

YARROW
Circulation problems (thrombosis, high blood pressure). Constipation, abdominal cramps, flatulence, and cystitis. Eczema, scar tissue, burns and cuts.
Calms hyperactivity.

YLANG YLANG
Respiratory conditions (rapid breathing). Rapid heart rate. Itchy skin, poor hair growth, insect bites.
Soothes excitable, stressed pets.

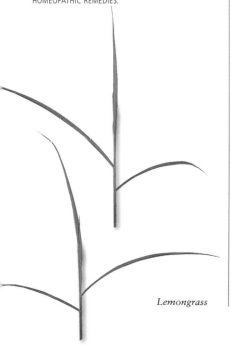
Lemongrass

Flower Remedies and Gem Essences

The history of flower remedies starts with Dr Edward Bach, who was originally a homeopath, working at the Royal London Homoeopathic Hospital. He noticed that people with similar personalities, moods, and attitudes to life tended to have similar ailments. He then discovered that essences of certain wild flowers and trees could correct any imbalance in personality and therefore treat any illness suffered by each "personality."

This link between physical illness and mental state is common throughout natural therapies – naturopathy treats the whole patient, not just the physical illness. Bach took this one stage further, demonstrating that if one addresses the mind, emotions, and spirit, the physical problems will automatically improve as a result.

In the 1920s and 1930s Bach identified the 38 flowers and trees that bear his name as the Bach Flower Remedies. Bach developed a process of harnessing the healing energy in each plant he used and preserving the resulting mixture.

Although developed for human patients, Bach Flower Remedies are equally applicable to pets. Anyone who has cared for a pet will realize how quickly we are able to pick up subtle changes in mood and disposition in pets. Mood and behavior changes often occur before physical symptoms of illness are evident. Alternatively, long-term physical disease may result in gradual changes in character and emotions. In both cases, flower remedies are important to consider as part of treatment for the patient. Other flower essences also exist – Australian Bush Flower and American flower essences.

In addition to flower remedies, gemstones have similar healing qualities. Centuries ago in India, gems were burned and their ash used as healing agents. Nowadays, gems are usually used as liquid essences; they are prepared in a similar way to flower essences, by harnessing and then preserving their healing qualities in alcohol.

Assessing the mood and behavior is of your pet is very important when selecting the appropriate flower or gem remedy.

ADMINISTERING FLOWER REMEDIES

- Administering flower and gem essences is relatively straightforward for pets.

- It is safe and effective to administer drops direct from the vial into the pet's mouth or beak.

- Take care not to let the dropper touch the tongue or lips. If it does so accidentally, rinse the dropper well immediately.

- If dosing by mouth is difficult, drops can be added to drinking water or to food if necessary. Often, the best results are obtained by oral dosing.

- Flower and gem essences are suitable for all pets, including birds. Even fish can be treated, by adding drops to the fish tank or pond. Where water is medicated, it is safe for unaffected pets to absorb

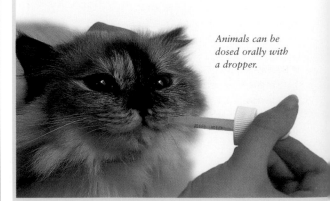

Animals can be dosed orally with a dropper.

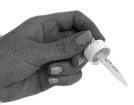

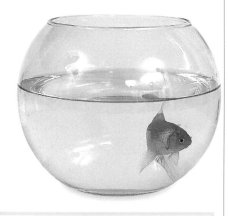

You can treat fish by adding flower remedies and gem essences to a bowl or tank. However, do not keep fish in bowls.

the remedies. If the healing energy of the remedy is not required, it will do no harm.

• The normal dose rate of flower and gem remedies for dogs and cats is one drop twice daily, and for all other pets one drop daily. Essences can be given for long periods safely, and often where problems are behavioral and emotional rather than physical, they need to be given for a month or more at a time.

• If the symptoms being treated are primarily physical, stop treatment as soon as the physical symptoms resolve.

• Because of the alcohol content, it is not wise to dose very small pets for long periods. Give for up to a week at a time, but stop using if any signs of inebriation occur!

BACH FLOWER REMEDIES

AGRIMONY
For pets that get upset by arguments and quarrels around them, and those that don't show outward signs of illness.

ASPEN
Pets that are generally fearful and anxious. Apprehensive when meeting strangers.

BEECH
Pets that overreact to little things.

CENTAURY
Pets that are easily dominated by other animals, and are over-anxious to please their owners.

CERATO
Pets that lack confidence, constantly looking at their owners for reassurance, and don't like being left on their own.

CHERRY PLUM
For stressed pets that sometimes snap or bite, but are then upset by what they have done.

CHESTNUT BUD
Pets that make the same mistakes over and over again.

CHICORY
Pets that like to rule the roost.

CLEMATIS
Pets that lack concentration and seem to live in a dream world. Often inactive, lacking in energy.

CRAB APPLE
A cleansing remedy, good to use during illness to remove toxins.

ELM
Pets that seem to be temporarily overwhelmed by life.

GENTIAN
Pets that are easily discouraged. Small things that happen upset them – for example, a short rainshower may put them off a walk completely.

GORSE
For pets that seem to have given in to illness, stop eating, and lose willpower.

HEATHER
For pets that will not leave you alone, always want your attention, and follow you everywhere, and may be destructive if left alone.

HOLLY
Pets that show signs of anger, hatred, and envy or jealousy. Useful for pets that dislike and may attack new pets (or people) introduced into the home.

HONEYSUCKLE
For homesickness; pets that try to return to their old home after a move, or are obviously unsettled in their new home, or get depressed when placed in boarding kennels.

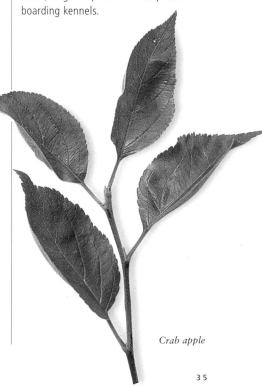

Crab apple

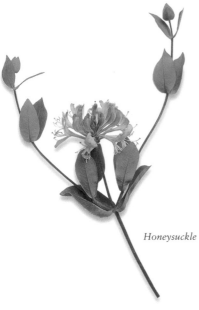

Honeysuckle

MIMULUS
For pets with a fear of something specific.
Any major phobia.

MUSTARD
For pets that get sudden spells of being miserable and depressed. Often the mood comes and goes.

OAK
Pets that are chronically unwell but keep going, though obviously struggling.

OLIVE
For post-viral weakness; the lack of energy and interest following an acute or long-term illness.

PINE
Pets that seem to take things personally; never seem quite satisfied with life.

RED CHESTNUT
Pets that are very worried by others being ill or upset around them.
Very anxious that things may go wrong, paranoid and sensitive.

ROCK ROSE
At times of panic, terror, and hysteria following an accident or shock.

ROCK WATER
Pets that are slaves to routine, following the same set patterns each day; obsessive-compulsive disorders.

Olive

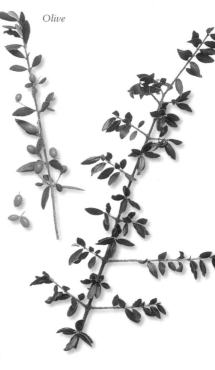

HORNBEAM
For lethargy and lack of energy, especially at the start of the day. A strengthening remedy during illness.

IMPATIENS
For impatient pets that want everything instantly. Hate being kept waiting.

LARCH
A remedy for lack of confidence.

Oak

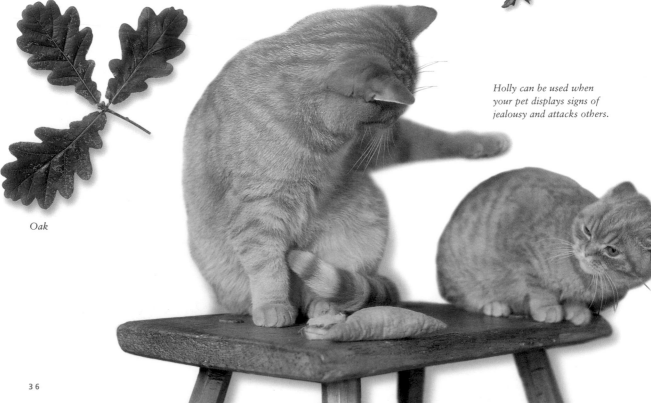

Holly can be used when your pet displays signs of jealousy and attacks others.

SCLERANTHUS
Pets that swing from one mood to another, whose energy levels go up and down. Helps travel-sick pets.

STAR OF BETHLEHEM
For grief, loss, and bereavement.

SWEET CHESTNUT
For when a pet just seems to have had enough. Useful for pets who hate traveling in cars.

VERVAIN
For disobedient pets that like things their own way.

VINE
Over-dominant pets.

WALNUT
Ideal for helping adjust to any changes life brings.

WATER VIOLET
The independent sort of pet that wants to be alone when ill; gentle but a little aloof or reserved.

WHITE CHESTNUT
For pets that can't get to sleep and seem to have thoughts and worries constantly going through their minds.

WILD OAT
Pets that seem dissatisfied, bored.

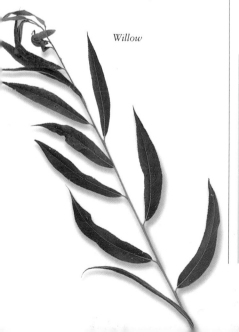
Willow

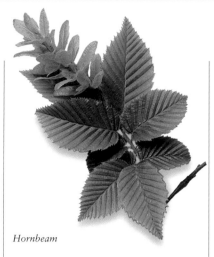
Hornbeam

WILD ROSE
Pets that seem indifferent to their fate, making little effort to recover even if not severely ill.

WILLOW
Pets that feel resentful and bitter.

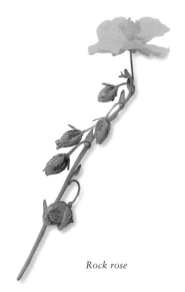
Rock rose

RESCUE REMEDY

A combination of Star of Bethlehem, for trauma and numbness; Rock Rose, for terror and panic; Impatiens, for irritability and tension; Cherry Plum for fear of losing control; and Clematis, for tendency to pass out.
It is an ideal remedy to use at the time of any accident or injury, shock or stressful situation.

GEM ESSENCES

CAT'S EYE
Nerve paralysis, cancer, joint disease.

CORAL
Warts and other skin growths.

DIAMOND
For epilepsy and urinary tract disorders.

EMERALD
Fevers and other inflammatory conditions.

ONYX
Liver disease, constipation, and loss of appetite.

PEARL
Respiratory problems – catarrh, bronchitis, asthma, kidney disease, and bladder stones.

RUBY
Anemia, joint disease (spondylosis, arthritis).

SAPPHIRE
For back pain, neuritis, asthma, and persistent bleeding.

TOPAZ
Thyroid imbalance, obesity, severe coughs, and glandular problems (pituitary, pancreatic, prostate, and adrenal).

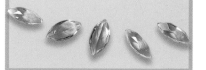

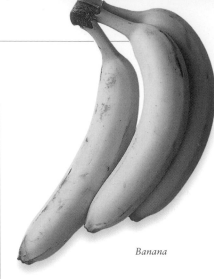

Banana

AUSTRALIAN BUSH AND AMERICAN FLOWER ESSENCES

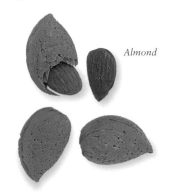

Almond

ALMOND
Rejuvenates and heals damaged tissues. Also helps immature pets to develop their full potential.

ALOE VERA
For behavioral problems brought on by stress.

AMARANTHUS
An immune system booster, ideal for weakened, debilitated animals.

APRICOT
Strengthens the body, especially when cancer is present.

AVOCADO
Improves absorption of materials in young animals.

BANANA
For food allergies, and to counteract the effects of food additives.

BELLS OF IRELAND
Rejuvenates older animals, helps those with symptoms of senility.

BLACK-EYED SUSAN
Hyperactive pets, often suffering restless sleep and irritable with colitis or other digestive problems.

BLUEBELL
Pets that have suffered emotional or physical abuse or deprivation. Useful for pets from rescue centers.

BORAGE
For elderly, chronically ill pets.

BOTTLEBRUSH
Improves acceptance of pets to other pets in the home.

BUSH FUCHSIA
Pets that lack concentration, find training difficult. They are intelligent, but are slow to learn.

CAMPHORA
Cleansing agent, helping at times of constipation and infections.

CELERY
For immune system balance; useful in auto-immune disease.

CAMOMILE
Dogs that will not stop barking, and for pets that get digestive upsets following emotional stress.

CHICAGO PEACE ROSE
Stabilizes nervous system (following injury, or in epileptics).

Hawthorne

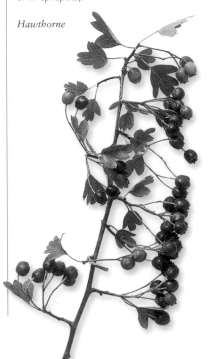

COMFREY
Regenerates nerves after injuries.

COSMOS
Helps training and obedience work by improving the pet–carer bond.
Also helps dogs at shows, in boarding kennels, or at training classes to have confidence when meeting another group of dogs.

COTTON
For mange and other skin disease.

CUCUMBER
For depression and lack of will power.

DILL
For arthritis, bony lumps and spurs, kidney stones, bladder stones.

GRAPEFRUIT
For injuries to head, neck, spine, and pelvis.

GRAY SPIDER FLOWER
For blind panic, immobilizing fear.

HAWTHORN
Cleansing remedy; useful for cataracts.

HELLEBORUS
For cancer and degenerative diseases of the elderly pet.

HIBBERTIA
Pets that never quite seem to be aware of their surroundings.

KANGAROO PAW
For clumsy pets, with shy and timid natures.

LUFFA
For skin allergies.

MANGO
Speeds healing after injuries.

MCCARTNEY ROSE
For immune system disease, especially leukemia.

MULLA MULLA
For the prevention and effects of sunburn, heat rashes, and exhaustion.

NASTURTIUM
Strengthens the nervous system; good for epilepsy and neuritis.

NYMPHENBERG ROSE
Strengthens the body during illness.

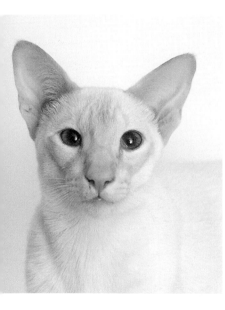

Prickly pear helps pets that are alone for long periods.

PANSY
For immune system diseases, especially when caused by virus infections.

PEACE ROSE
Gives courage to face illness and adversity.

PEACH
Helps pets that absorb emotional stresses from their carers.

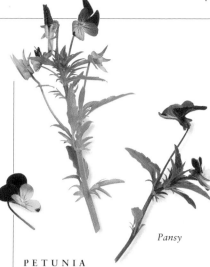

Pansy

PETUNIA
For pets with repeated bad habits or disobedience; helps them respond to training classes.

PIMPERNEL
For unusual behavior patterns and nervous disease in general, twitching heads or limbs in particular.

PRICKLY PEAR
For pets that have to be left alone for long periods, to help them adjust and be patient.

REDWOOD
For kidney and bladder diseases.

SAGE
A circulatory essence for heart disease, retained fluid, heart coughs.

ST JOHN'S WORT
A natural painkiller, and helps relieve fear and anxiety.

SALVIA
Helps restore emotional balance in stressful experiences.

SNAPDRAGON
For pets that chew things or lick themselves repeatedly, and mouth-oriented problems of this nature.

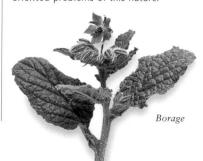

Borage

STAR TULIP
For hypersensitivity and allergies, especially with hair loss.

STURT DESERT ROSE
Pets that seem to feel guilty even when things aren't their fault.

SUGAR BEET
For diabetes and pancreatic conditions, and the cataracts that can accompany diabetes.

SUNFLOWER
For heatstroke, sunburn, or any ill effects of heat or sunshine.

SWEET FLAG
Given before a move or a long journey. Reduces fear and anxiety.

TIGER LILY
For aggression, biting, scratching, hostility of any kind.

TOMATO
Cleansing remedy, for catarrh, all kinds of discharges, blood poisoning.

Sunflower

WARATAH
Good at times of emotional crisis, sudden bereavement, and stress.

WEDDING BUSH
For pets that seem aloof and distant, or those that tend to run off and seem to want to escape the confines of the home.

WHITE LIGHTNIN' ROSE
Speedy healing for wounds, cuts, and burns.

WOOD BETONY
Improves recovery rate after operations – ideal to give before neutering operation.

ZUCCHINI
For convalescence after illness; builds up health and strength.

Herbal Medicine

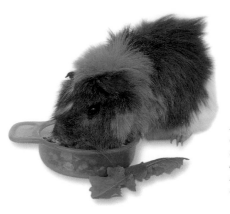

Herbal medicine is probably the oldest system of medicine in the world. Nothing could be more natural than to discover and use the healing powers of the herbs and flowers around us to cure ourselves – and our animals. In fact, animals in the wild have an innate ability to seek out and eat the herbs that will help them when they are ill or injured.

Modern drugs were originally extracts of herbs, but nowadays are usually synthesized variants of isolated chemicals found in those herbs, rather than the whole plant.

Herbal medicines themselves are gentler, safer, and often more effective than their conventional chemical equivalents or derivatives, because the whole plant, or a large part of it, is used. As with most kinds of natural medicines, this means that the whole body is treated, not just the particular physical symptoms. This has a greater all-round benefit to the patient. It also reduces the risk of side-effects. However, any herb given in overdose can cause an adverse reaction; as with all natural medicines, herbs are safe only when prepared and used correctly.

Adding fresh or dried herbs to food is an ancient and safe method of healing.

Herbal medicines can be administered in many different ways:

• As the fresh herb – leaves and stems can be chopped and mixed with food. For instance, feverfew grows in many gardens and is a good anti-arthritic agent – the leaves can be added to the diet. Dandelion leaves can be added to the diet for a natural diuretic action.

• As proprietary powders and tablets, tinctures, and lotions. Many pet shops, health food shops, and pharmacies now stock herbal remedies for pets in this form, or you can buy them by mail order.

• As the dried herb added to food. A little effectiveness may be lost when herbs are dried, but fresh herbs are rarely available on a regular basis, and dried herbs make a very good substitute.

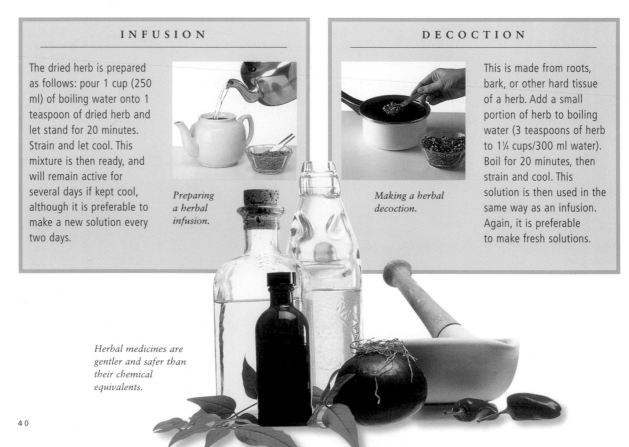

INFUSION

The dried herb is prepared as follows: pour 1 cup (250 ml) of boiling water onto 1 teaspoon of dried herb and let stand for 20 minutes. Strain and let cool. This mixture is then ready, and will remain active for several days if kept cool, although it is preferable to make a new solution every two days.

Preparing a herbal infusion.

DECOCTION

This is made from roots, bark, or other hard tissue of a herb. Add a small portion of herb to boiling water (3 teaspoons of herb to 1¼ cups/300 ml water). Boil for 20 minutes, then strain and cool. This solution is then used in the same way as an infusion. Again, it is preferable to make fresh solutions.

Making a herbal decoction.

Herbal medicines are gentler and safer than their chemical equivalents.

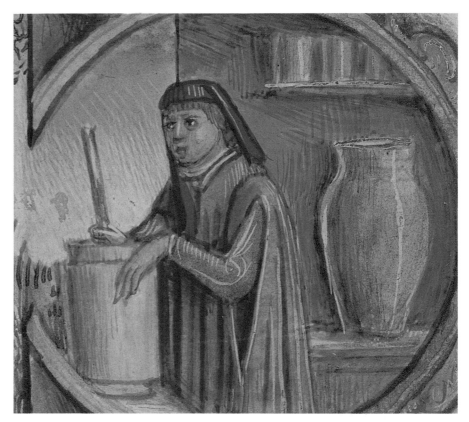

In medieval times, monks would prepare and administer herbal remedies.

• As an eye wash. Make up herb as an infusion. Add a pinch of salt, then strain through unbleached filter paper to maintain purity.

• As an oil infusion. Cover 3 teaspoons of dried herb with 1 cup (250 ml) of pure vegetable oil, then simmer in a water bath (direct heat might burn the oil). Simmer for two hours. Strain again and let cool, then the mixture is ready for use. Oil infusions can be massaged into the skin or fur, and rubbed over stiff joints and sore muscles.

HERBAL TREATMENT

Herbal treatment is suitable for most pets except fish. Proprietary preparations will come with dosage directions printed on the label.

Fresh and dried herbs should be added to the diet in small amounts – two or three leaves per day for a dog, one for a cat, and one every two to three days for smaller pets. Do not dose with any herb for more than a month without a break, to ensure that overdosage cannot occur.

Infusions and decoctions should be given as follows – 2–4 teaspoons twice daily for a dog, 2 teaspoons twice daily for a cat, 1 teaspoon daily for a rabbit, ½ teaspoon daily for smaller pets. Dosing pets with liquids can be difficult, but a dropper or small syringe can be used, making the process practicable in most cases. A week's course should be sufficient for acute problems, a month for more chronic, long-term problems.

Eyewashes should be used twice daily until symptoms resolve. An eye bath can be used, or a dropper to drop the lotion into the eye, or cotton wool can be soaked with the infusion and this can be squeezed into the eye. Any utensils used should be sterilized before use, as they may come into contact with the eye and become contaminated.

Oil infusions should be massaged in once or twice daily until symptoms resolve.

Additionally, herbs are sometimes used in the form of creams and ointments, compresses (for swollen joints), in poultices (for drawing infection from wounds and abscesses), and as shampoos.

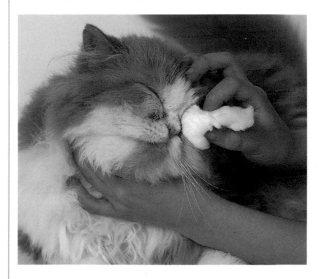

A herbal infusion or decoction can be used twice daily as an effective eye wash.

HERBS FOR USE IN PETS

The following herbs are thirty of the most commonly used and are safe, effective animal remedies.

BARBERRY

Mainly a liver remedy, acting as a tonic and stimulating bile flow.
Good digestive stabilizer, relieves constipation, improves appetite, helpful when the spleen is enlarged.

YARROW

An anti-inflammatory herb, beneficial for arthritis, the early stage of fevers, aches and pains in general, diarrhea, and colitis. It is supportive for pets undergoing radiotherapy.

BEARBERRY (UVA URSI)

Acts mainly on the urinary tract. Used to treat cystitis, especially in combination with marshmallow. Beneficial for chronic kidney failure, bladder stones, urinary incontinence.

LADY'S MANTLE

Acts particularly on the uterus. Beneficial for bleeding from the uterus, hormonal imbalance, for infertility.
DO NOT GIVE DURING PREGNANCY.

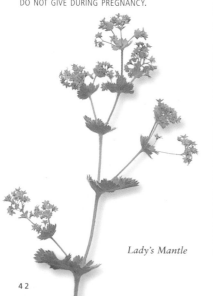

Lady's Mantle

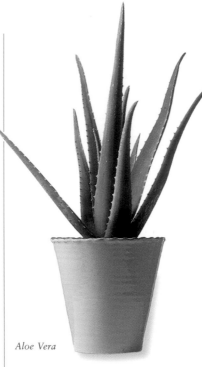

Aloe Vera

BUCHU

A diuretic and urinary tract stimulant. Specific for chronic cystitis, bladder weakness and incontinence, bladder stones, chronic kidney disease, enlarged prostate glands.

ALOE VERA

Apply the gel from a cut leaf to burns, sunburn, infected cuts, eczema, dry, itchy skin, and ringworm to obtain rapid healing. Can be taken internally as a general tonic.

CALIFORNIAN BUCKTHORN (CASCARA)

A natural laxative. Ideal for constipation. Improves appetite and is a general tonic for the digestive tract. Give for short periods only – two or three days at the most.

MARSHMALLOW

An anti-irritant – good for irritable bladder (especially in combination with yarrow) and irritable bowel conditions. Also treats dry, non-productive coughs.

CAYENNE (CAPSICUM)

A tonic, stimulating herb. Improves circulation, especially to the kidneys, so used for a variety of heart, circulatory,

and kidney conditions. Improves appetite and digestion.

BURDOCK

A liver and skin remedy. Supports the liver when diseased, especially in combination with dandelion. Good for eruptive skin conditions – rashes, pyoderma (infection of the skin), abscesses.

DANDELION

One of the oldest medicinal herbs. A cleansing, detoxifying herb. The leaves are used as a diuretic to help clear fluid retention. The root is good for liver problems and jaundice, skin eruptions, fur loss, and anal gland problems.

MARIGOLD

Healing and anti-inflammatory. Available in lotions and creams for itchy, sore skin, and for rashes, grazes, cuts, and fungal skin infections. As an infusion, good for digestive upsets and ulcers.

ELDERBERRY

Blood purifier, treats anemia. Stomach and liver problems will also respond to elderberry. It also has a natural diuretic action. Improves skin pigmentation.

CAMOMILE

Camomile tea settles digestive upsets – flatulence, colic, and colitis. Also for troublesome teething in puppies and kittens.

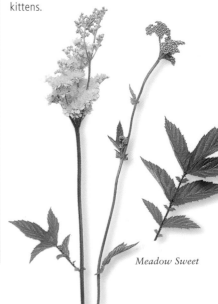

Meadow Sweet

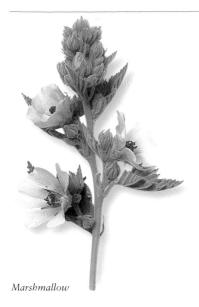

Marshmallow

EUCALYPTUS
Especially useful for chest problems –
bronchitis, catarrh, sinusitis. Apply locally
to the skin to treat ringworm. Also a
cystitis remedy.

HAWTHORN
The berries and flowers are used to
produce this herbal support for heart
conditions; often taken in the form of
a tincture.

GARLIC
Important and versatile herb. Antiviral,
antifungal, antibacterial, and
antiparasitic. It tones the circulation,
helping reduce the risk of strokes in
older animals. It is widely used to treat
infection of all kinds, and as a preventive
against worm and flea infestations, to
treat sinusitis and catarrh, and in the
management of diabetes. Give a break
from treatment now and again if giving
long term.

ECHINACEA
Excellent immune system booster. Ideal
for patients with known or suspected
immune system defects. Helps prevent,
and treat repeated skin infections.
Available as tablets and tinctures.

GENTIAN
A digestive tonic, good for chronic
digestive conditions. Also a calming
agent – suitable to treat nervous and
hysterical pets. Has the disadvantage
of a very bitter taste.

MEADOW SWEET
For diarrhea in hot weather, general
digestion upsets and flatulence, clear
sandy mineral deposits in urine, helpful
for arthritis.

HOPS
A soothing, calming remedy. Good for
anxiety and restlessness, sleeplessness,
epilepsy, and hyperactivity. Also improves
appetite, and aids colic and digestive
upsets. Not advisable to give in the
usual form humans
take it – that is,
in beer!

FENNEL
A soothing herb. Excellent for irritable
bowel disease and flatulence. An
antidepressant, acting as a tonic to the
nervous system. Also promotes milk flow
in nursing pets.

JUNIPER
The berries are used to produce an
excellent cystitis remedy, whether acute
or chronic. Juniper decoction can be
brushed onto the coat to help repel
fleas, lice, and ticks.

GINKGO
Has tonic effect on the circulation.
Especially helpful for elderly pets with
symptoms of senility – it improves blood
flow to the brain. Sometimes slows down
hearing loss in older pets. Reduces
likelihood of strokes in old animals.
Improves memory.

KAVA KAVA
An unusual remedy from the South Sea
islands (rumored to be hallucinogenic).
No such effects known in pets, where it
is a good remedy for cystitis, vaginal
infections, and prostate problems.

DEVIL'S CLAW
An excellent anti-inflammatory herb for
joint and back problems.
Relieves arthritis, spondylitis, and
osteoarthritis symptoms. Can help calm
and restore itchy skins that seem to have
no obvious cause.

LICORICE
Licorice root is soothing and anti-
inflammatory. Good for irritable bowel
syndrome, ulcers, and persistent bowel
infections. Also for irritable dry coughs.
Large or continual doses may be
laxative.

*Gingko boosts energy and circulation.
It is especially benefical for elderly or
senile animals.*

WITCH HAZEL
Used externally as an excellent healing
agent for bruises, cuts, and wounds. As a
compress for sprains, swollen joints, and
sunburn. As an eyewash for sore eyes.

NETTLES
Stinging nettles – although not a favourite
herb to collect – are ideal for treating
eczema, cystitis, bladder stones and
sediment, anemia, chronic kidney disease,
and arthritis.
Such a humble plant is nevertheless
a powerful herb.

ST JOHN'S WORT
Often called the herbal Prozac, it is
an effective and safe antidepressant.
A good painkiller, particularly for
chronic back problems and in cases
of neuritis.

Homeopathy

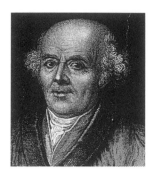

Dr Samuel Hahnemann

In the late eighteenth century, a German doctor called Samuel Hahnemann developed a system of medicine that he named homeopathy. The term homeopathy comes from the Greek, meaning "similar suffering." The term reflects the key principle behind homeopathy: that a substance of mineral, plant, or animal origin which causes adverse symptoms in an individual could cure those same symptoms when given in a minute homeopathic dose.

Between 1790 and 1805 Hahnemann tested 60 drugs from a variety of sources on himself and a small group of students. This method of "proving" substances to discover the range of symptoms they were capable of causing enabled Hahnemann to find out what they could also cure. There are now over 3,000 homeopathic remedies, all produced by diluting the original substance in several stages, and by shaking, or "succussing", the solution at each dilution to add energy to the product. This system of increasingly diluting but also energizing the starting material produces remedies that are so dilute as to be completely safe and free from side-effects, yet are powerful enough to act as strong healing agents.

TREATING THE INDIVIDUAL

It was also found that homeopathic remedies corresponded to the mental and emotional states of a patient.

The idea of a homeopathic "constitution" – that is, the concept that each individual (person or animal) is a particular physical, mental, and emotional type and will correspond to a particular homeopathic remedy – is

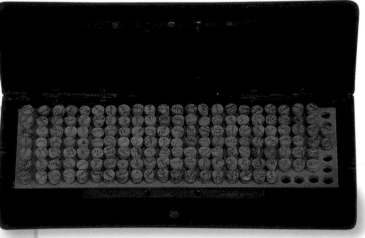

Available in several different forms and varying potencies, homeopathic remedies will treat almost all diseases found in pets.

especially useful when dealing with chronic and deep-seated disease. Homeopathy can be used to treat almost all diseases found in pets, but it is especially effective for chronic conditions such as skin disorders, arthritis, and long-standing respiratory problems.

Remedies are also produced in different potencies. The commonly available potency is known as 6c, and this will be marked on the tablet container. The correct remedy for a condition will be effective in any potency, but the higher the potency (the larger the number before the "c") the

TREATMENT

The remedies are available as tablets, powders, granules, pillules, liquids, and ointments. The dosage rates are as follows:

• For acute conditions, give one tablet every 15 minutes for three hours, then one tablet hourly for the rest of the day. After this, give one tablet three times daily for three more days, or until all symptoms have disappeared.

• For chronic conditions, give one tablet three times daily for one week, followed by one tablet twice daily for three weeks.

• If other forms of remedy are used, the equivalent doses are: one tablet = one powder = 12 granules/pillules = 3 drops of liquid.

• Ointments are normally added twice daily to the affected area of skin.

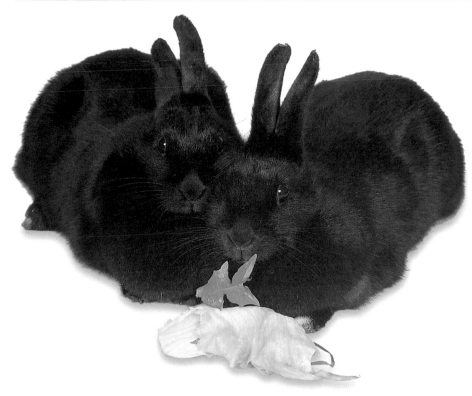

If an animal will not take a tablet whole, the homeopathic remedy can be administered as a crushed powder sprinkled over food.

greater the healing action will be. However, homeopathy works on the principle of minimum dosage – only give the amount necessary to initiate healing. If too high a potency is given, the symptoms may temporarily become aggravated, so you should use 6c potencies only (unless advised otherwise by a vet with expertise in homeopathy).

GIVING A REMEDY

Homeopathic remedies should be given by mouth, if possible. This should be done away from food and without touching the tablets, as their effectiveness can be reduced by certain chemicals in foodstuffs and even by traces of chemicals on fingers. Tablets do not need to be swallowed;

they are more effective if allowed to dissolve and be absorbed from the lining of the mouth. For pets that will not take tablets by mouth, tablets may be crushed and mixed with a small amount of bland food – butter for a cat, lettuce for a rabbit or tortoise, and so on. For fish, tablets may simply be dissolved in their water.

Care must be taken when storing homeopathic remedies. Keep some away from strong smells, bright light, and excessive heat or cold. Magnetic fields from electrical equipment can also render the medicines less effective. Although this advice makes homeopathic products sound very fragile, they will remain active for years if stored correctly.

POWERFUL AROMAS

Herbs or foodstuffs with powerful aromas – such as garlic – may also reduce the potency of homeopathic remedies, and should not be given at the same time. Some essential oils – such as peppermint – may also reduce the effectiveness of homeopathic remedies.

Garlic

Homeopathic remedies are more effective when dissolved in the mouth.

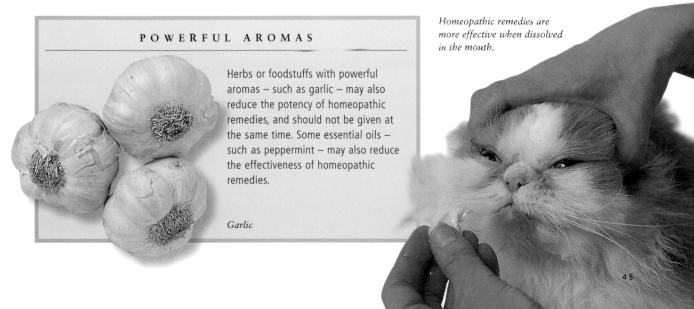

TOP 75 HOMEOPATHIC REMEDIES

ACID. NIT.
(NITRIC ACID)

Treats blisters and ulcers in the mouth, warts that bleed easily, liver and kidney problems. Particularly good for ulceration where moist skin meets dry skin – lips, nostrils, anus.

ACID SAL.
(SALICYLIC ACID)

An anti-inflammatory, treating pain and stiffness, especially in small joints – toes, wrist, and ankle joints. Also for retinal hemorrhage in the eye, sore throats, and mouth ulcers.

ACONITE (MONKSHOOD)

Treats shock, especially after operations or exposure to cold winds or dry heat. Ideal at the start of any fever. Good for sore eyes and nosebleeds. Patient is usually thirsty.

AGNUS CASTUS
(BERRIES OF THE PLANT)

Treats reproductive and hormonal problems – infertility, vaginal discharges, failure of testicles to drop in male animals, retained afterbirths. Also mouth ulcers and enlarged spleen.

ALLIUM CEPA
(RED ONION)

Cut an onion and what happens? Runny eyes, runny nose – so the homeopathic onion remedy cures those symptoms. Colds and flu infections, watery eye discharges, and allergies causing hay fever-like symptoms.

ALOE
(SOCOTRINE ALOES)

Combats excessive use of conventional drugs. Useful to give after a long course of drugs has been administered, especially if liver problems or bowel conditions are a feature.

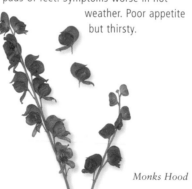

Honeybee

ANT. CRUD. (BLACK ANTIMONYSULPHIDE)

Treats eczema – especially where the skin is dry and scabs form, under which is a sticky secretion. Warty growths on pads of feet. Symptoms worse in hot weather. Poor appetite but thirsty.

Monks Hood

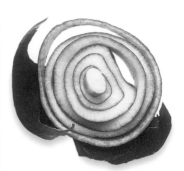

Red Onion

ANT. TART.
(TARTAR EMETIC)

Treats respiratory problems – mucus can be heard rattling in chest, but little is coughed up. Breathing may be difficult. Good for bronchitis, pneumonia, emphysema.

APIS MEL.
(HONEY BEE)

Treats stings and bites, tissue swelling, swollen joints; also acute kidney disease. Patient is worse for heat, and not thirsty.

ARNICA
(LEOPARD'S BANE)

TOP TEN REMEDY

If you only ever use one homeopathic remedy, use Arnica. It is the single most useful remedy in the homeopathic repertoire. Any trauma will respond to it – bruising, injury, hemorrhage, tissue damage of any kind. It reduces shock (often given with Aconite) – ideal to give to pets after giving birth. Can be used as

Arnica is an excellent treatment after the trauma of giving birth. It reduces shock and aids recovery.

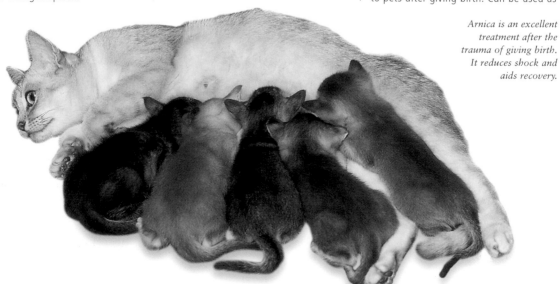

cream or ointment to apply to bruised muscles and tendons (do not apply to broken skin). Good for bleeding within the eye and helps failing hearts. Always remember Arnica as *the* injury remedy and keep the cream or ointment available.

ARSEN. ALB. (ARSENIC TRIOXIDE)
TOP TEN REMEDY

Wide-acting remedy. Treats dry eczema, with scurfy skin and hair loss. Vomiting and diarrhea, especially when caused by food poisoning. Conjunctivitis with acrid discharge. Coughing and wheezing. Canine distemper. Feline infectious enteritis. The patient who needs Arsen. alb. will be very restless, need warmth, and tend to be thirsty – but will drink only small amounts at a time. Symptoms are usually worse toward midnight. Always remember, and keep available, Arsen. alb. for sudden acute attacks of gastroenteritis – and as a remedy for restlessness.

BELLADONNA (DEADLY NIGHTSHADE)

Treats fevers and inflammations. Acute infections, heatstroke, mastitis, hot swollen joints, inflamed skin, and sore throats. Pupils are often dilated, the patient is sensitive to touch, and is often thirsty.

BELLIS PER. (DAISY)

Treats bruising, sprains, strains. Especially good for deep muscular bruising – pelvic injuries after accidents, or giving birth. Patient is too stiff to move. Hemorrhage under the skin.

BORAX (SODIUM BIBORATE)

Treats blisters and ulcers of the mouth and feet, and sore eyes, helping to treat inturning eyelids (entropion). Patients

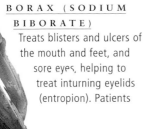

Belladona

are very nervous, and often have a fear of downward movement. Nails and claws may become loose.

BOVISTA (PUFFBALL)

Treats eczema, particularly eczema of the head area. Severe itching of the face – patient rubs face against objects. Skin thickened and inflamed and bleeds easily. Skin is moist, then becomes crusty.

BUFO (TOAD POISON)

Treats skin and nervous system diseases. Epilepsy, nervousness, fear of other animals, behavior problems. Infections in skin – abscesses, repeated infections of the toes and feet. Also for nodules in mammary glands.

CALC.CARB. (OYSTER SHELL)
TOP TEN REMEDY

A major remedy for bone and joint problems. Arthritis and stiffness; abnormalities of bones in young growing animals. Eye problems, especially cataracts, chronic catarrh, enlarged lymph glands. Skin problems with a tendency to warts. Teeth may be late in appearing in young animals, and milk teeth may be retained for long periods. The patient who needs calc. carb. tends to be overweight, inactive, need warmth and comfort, and dislike cold weather and being bathed. Often greedy. Remember as the big and bony remedy.

CALC. PHOS. (PHOSPHATE OF LIME)

A remedy for bone problems. Brittle or weak bones, abnormal skeletal development in young animals, arthritis in older pets.
Like Calc. carb., the patient is better for warmth and hates cold and damp; but is lean and active, not overweight.

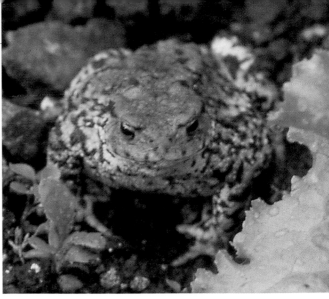

Derived from the common toad, the homeopathic remedy Bufo treats skin infections and nervous system diseases.

CALC. SULPH. (PLASTER OF PARIS)

Treats persistently discharging, purulent wounds or ulcers which are slow to heal. Creamy or yellow discharge. Good for discharging abscesses in rabbits in particular. Chronic catarrh and sinusitis.

CANTHARIS (SPANISH FLY)
TOP TEN REMEDY

A major remedy for burning pains. It is the classic treatment for cystitis. If started as soon as symptoms appear, it will almost always stop cystitis developing. Symptoms are frequency of passing urine, pain on passing urine, blood in urine, small amounts of urine passed. Any condition accompanied by a burning pain will respond to Cantharis – burns and scalds themselves, acute eczema with constant itching, painful insect bites and stings, and acute gastroenteritis where there is straining and passing blood. Painful areas are relieved by rubbing, but are sensitive to touch. Remember Cantharis as the burning remedy.

CARBO. VEG. (CHARCOAL)

Known in homeopathic circles as the corpse reviver, Carbo. veg. treats shock and collapse from all causes. Patient often needs air, despite feeling cold. Also good for flatulence and colic.

CAULOPHYLLUM
(BLUE COHOSH)
Known as the squaw root, because Native American women used it as an aid to an easy birth. Caulophyllum given regularly during pregnancy improves the tone of the uterus muscles, and reduces the likelihood of problems at birth. This remedy is also good for pains in small joints.

CAMOMILE
(CAMOMILE PLANT)
Mainly known as a remedy for teething pains in young pets (or human babies), often accompanied by greenish diarrhea, sore eyes and ears, enlarged lymph glands, and of course red, sore gums.

CHINA (OR CINCHONA)
(PERUVIAN BARK)
The first remedy discovered by Hahnemann, as a treatment for malaria. Good for all fevers that cause weakness, when temperature keeps going up and down, and dehydration is a feature. Patients want warmth and fresh air.

COCCULUS
(INDIAN COCKLE)
Treats nervous system disease. Epilepsy, and brain damage, especially if there is difficulty in opening the mouth and in swallowing. Symptoms worsen during prolonged movement. A good travel sickness remedy.

COFFEA CRUDA
(UNROASTED COFFEE)
Drinking coffee, which contains caffeine, keeps you awake, so homeopathic coffee relieves symptoms of restlessness or sleeplessness – especially in the early hours of the morning. Old pets that wake frequently at night respond well to this remedy.

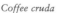

Coffee cruda

DIGITALIS (FOXGLOVE)
Treats heart conditions displaying a weak, slow, irregular pulse. Heart is enlarged and thin-walled. Fluid retention occurs. Patient may suffer black-outs on exertion, and tongue may turn blue.

DROSERA (SUNDEW)
A remedy for coughing. Spasmodic, dull cough, with retching or even vomiting. Frequent bouts of coughing, which may sound as if something is caught in the throat. Symptoms become worse when the patient is excited.

EUPHRASIA (EYEBRIGHT)
As its common name suggests, an eye remedy. For conjunctivitis, with much sticky, mucoid, catarrhal discharge. Sensitivity to light. Used internally but also as eye drops.

FERRUM MET. (IRON)
Treats anemia – any condition where anemia is a symptom will respond, especially in young animals. Often a poor appetite alternates with great hunger. This remedy is good for accelerating recovery after parasitic infections.

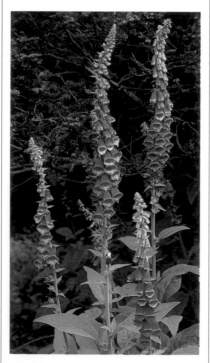

Digitalis purpurea (Foxglove)

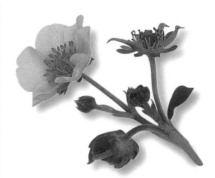

Frageria vesca (Wild strawberry)

FERRUM PHOS.
(IRON PHOSPHATE)
Good for the early stages of fevers. Patient is hot, often with inflammation of eyes and ears. Nosebleeds may occur, gums and lips look reddened, joints may be stiff and swollen.

FRAGARIA VESCA
(WILD STRAWBERRY)
Main use of fragaria is to help prevent or slow down the build-up of tartar and plaque on teeth. Given regularly (twice a day for three days each month) it can reduce the need for a toothbrush!

GELSEMIUM
(YELLOW JASMINE)
A remedy for the weak animal – weakness following persistent infections such as cat flu. Also a good anxiety remedy – fear of noise, fear of other animals. Patient often rigid with fear; rooted to the spot and trembling.

GRAPHITES
(BLACK LEAD)
Primarily a skin remedy. Dry, itchy skin with excessive molting. Skin smells unpleasant. Folds of skin may become filled with a sticky discharge. Patient likes warmth, but this makes the skin condition worse.

HAMAMELIS
(WITCH HAZEL)
A remedy for hemorrhage, in particular of dark, thick blood, which clots poorly. Good for ear hematomas. Speeds up reabsorption of blood clots.

HEPAR. SULPH.
(CALCIUM SULPHIDE)
A major remedy for treating pus. Abscesses, infected cysts, ear infections, purulent eye discharge, infected ulcers. Can be given as a preventive following bites to prevent infection. Patient is sensitive to touch, better for warmth.

HYDRASTIS
(GOLDEN SEAL)
Suits thick, yellow catarrh and secretions, especially from eyes, ears, or vagina. Good for mammary and other tumors. Also a remedy to support liver conditions.

HYPERICUM
(ST JOHN'S WORT)
A pain-relieving remedy, particularly pain at nerve endings – lacerated wounds; toe, tail, and ear injuries. Helps reduce post-operative pain, and the pain of spinal conditions, such as slipped discs.

IGNATIA
(ST IGNATIUS' BEAN)
Treats nervous and behavioral disorders, grief, and bereavement. Pets that hate being alone. Also epileptic and highly strung pets .

IPECAC.
(IPECACUANHA ROOT)
Treats persistent vomiting, often accompanied by a spasmodic cough. Nose bleeds with bright red blood occurring intermittently. Vomiting after operations.

KALI. BICH. (POTASSIUM BICHROMATE)
Treats yellow, stringy discharges, especially from eyes and nose. Vomiting yellow fluid, or brown frothy diarrhea. Symptoms worse in mornings and in hot weather.

St John's Wort

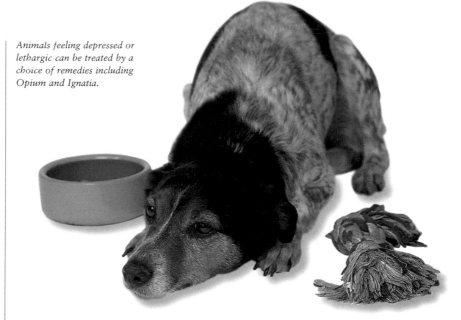

Animals feeling depressed or lethargic can be treated by a choice of remedies including Opium and Ignatia.

LEDUM (MARSH TEA)
A natural antitetanus remedy. Give after a puncture wound with Hypericum to relieve pain. Skin around wound is bluish and cold.

LEMNA MINOR
(DUCKWEED)
Treats sinusitis and catarrh. Often the discharge is an infected mucoidal catarrh, and bloodstained.

LYCOPODIUM
(CLUB MOSS)
TOP TEN REMEDY
Beneficial for liver and kidneys in particular. Tendency to a build-up of gas in the bowels; patient is prone to persistent digestive upsets. Patient eats well, but can manage only small amounts at a time; usually thin. Often passes red sediment in urine. Suits pets that are cautious and dislike being left alone.

MAG. PHOS.(MAGNESIUM PHOSPHATE)
An anticramp remedy. Painful muscles, often with twitching or trembling of legs. Old pets who are weak and tend to fall forward.

MERC. CORR.(CORROSIVE SUBLIMATE OF MERCURY)
For corrosive symptoms – sore ears with green discharge, conjunctivitis with burning tears, mouth ulcers with thick saliva, painful diarrhea, kidney disease with great thirst.

MERC. SOL. (MERCURY)
The less acute version of Merc. corr. Similar conditions – diarrhea, kidney problems, eye and ear conditions of a milder nature. Good for wet eczema.

MEZEREUM
(SPRING OLIVE)
Mainly used for eczema, especially of the face and head. Skin has crusty scabs, surrounded by a red area. Under the scab is thick purulent discharge.

NATRUM MUR.
(SODIUM CHLORIDE)
An excellent homeopathic remedy for kidney disease with great thirst, dry skin, sometimes watery eyes and nose, loss of weight, and anemia.

NUX VOMICA
(POISON NUT)
TOP TEN REMEDY
Primarily a digestive and liver remedy. It helps detoxify and remove ill effects of poisons, toxins, and conventional drugs from the system. Often given to clear the system before the main homeopathic remedy is started. Exceptionally good to relieve digestive upsets after pets have eaten too much or unsuitable foods. Also

good for pets with digestive problems after operations – lack of appetite, or constipation. Patients that need nux vomica tend to be a little irritable, dislike too much noise, feel better after resting or in damp weather. Remember it as the clearing remedy.

OPIUM
(OPIUM POPPY)

As Opium use causes constipation, so homeopathic Opium is an excellent remedy for persistent constipation. Also for any condition with lethargy, weakness, or paralysis.

ORNITHOGALUM
(STAR OF BETHLEHEM)

Treats stomach complaints, especially vomiting caused by a condition known as pyloric stenosis. Beneficial for stomach cancer.

PETROLEUM (OIL)

Good for eczema, with dry, cracked, red, and raw bleeding skin; symptoms are worse in damp weather, better when warm and dry. Also travel sickness.

PHOSPHORUS

Top Ten Remedy

Treats degenerative conditions. Suits liver, bone, pancreatic, and kidney disease. Jaundice may be present. Also for painful coughs, wounds that bleed easily and will not stop, ulcerated

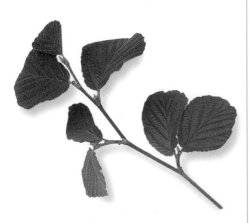

Witch Hazel

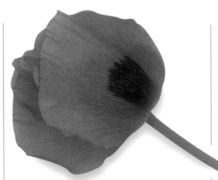

Opium poppy

bleeding gums, colitis with mucus and blood, tendency to vomit food shortly after eating. Symptoms tend to appear suddenly. The patient reacts violently to sudden noises – such as thunder, and fireworks. Patients tend to be thin and in poor condition, hyperactive, and nervous. Symptoms are better in cool conditions and after rest. Remember it as the degenerative remedy.

PODOPHYLLUM
(MAY APPLE)

Mainly a diarrhea remedy. Keynote is colicky pain, vomiting of bile, and particularly an explosive diarrhea with greenish, watery faeces, but no pain or straining.

PSORINUM
(SCABIES VESICLE)

A good mange remedy, and any skin condition with a dull and smelly coat, and the patient loses heat.

PULSATILLA
(WIND ANEMONE)

Top Ten Remedy

Often known as the female remedy, helping many female hormone imbalances such as infertility, false pregnancy, and uterine infection – bland, creamy mucus from nose, eyes, vagina. Also an excellent remedy for catarrh. Patients are frequently shy and often have alternating symptoms – constipation one day, diarrhea the next. Patients dislike heat, but love the open air. Remember it as the catarrh and hormonal remedy.

RHUS TOX.(POISON IVY)

° Top Ten Remedy °

The best known homeopathic anti-inflammatory remedy. Relieves the inflammation and pain of arthritis, conjunctivitis, otitis, and eczema. Redness, soreness, and itching are common signs. Symptoms are better for movement, worse for rest, and worst of all on first movement after resting. Damp, cold weather makes symptoms worse. Remember it as the inflammation remedy.

RUTA GRAV. (RUE)

Treats tendon and ligament damage – sprains, strains, and cartilage injuries. Also good for red, sore eyes and bowel incontinence.

SCUTELLARIA
(SKULLCAP)

A calming remedy for hysteria, hyperactivity, epilepsy, and unusual behavior patterns.

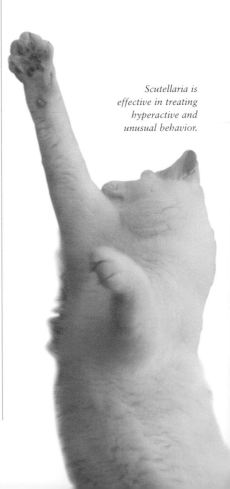

Scutellaria is effective in treating hyperactive and unusual behavior.

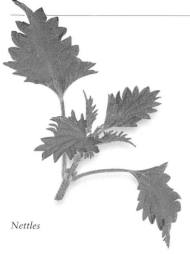

Nettles

SECALE (RYE FUNGUS)
Improves circulation to damaged tissue –
for instance, caged birds, when blood
flow is obstructed by a tight leg band.
Also for uterine disease.

SEPIA (CUTTLEFISH INK)
A female hormone balancing remedy for
infertility, false pregnancy, pyometra. Also
for circular skin lesions such as ringworm.
Patients are often moody and bad-
tempered.

SILICEA (FLINT)
Helps push unwanted foreign materials
(grass seeds, splinters) from the body.
Also shrinks scar tissue and chronic
inflammatory tissue, and heals chronically
infected tissue.

SPONGIA TOSTA (ROASTED SPONGE)
Valuable as a remedy for the coughing
that often accompanies heart disease –
congested lungs, cough worse for
exercise.

STAPHISAGRIA (STAVESACRE)
For cystitis, sore eyes, and complications
following operations. Also a remedy for
resentment, such as animals that are
upset by the introduction of a new pet.

SULFUR (SULPHUR)
TOP TEN REMEDY
A major remedy for skin problems,
especially mange. Skin is dry, dirty
looking, reddened and smelly with
intense itching, and hot to the touch.
Patients that need sulfur are often
overweight and stubborn. They dislike
heat and may lie on cold surfaces. They
need open air, and may have breathing
problems when inside. Like Nux vomica,
can be used as a clearing remedy.
Remember it as the hot, itchy remedy.

SYZYGIUM (JAMBOL SEED)
A specific remedy in the treatment of
diabetes. Using Syzygium means insulin
doses can be reduced, or sometimes
eliminated.

TARENTULA HISP. (SPANISH SPIDER)
A useful remedy for epilepsy and other
nervous system diseases. Head shaking is
often a symptom.

THLASPI BURSA (SHEPHERD'S PURSE)
For cystitis and other bladder problems.
Relieves the build up of sandy sediment
and bladder stones. Urine may be
bloodstained.

THUJA (ARBOR VITAE)
Treats growths, especially warts and
cysts. Anal tumors often respond. Useful
to give at vaccination time as a
protection against side-effects.

URANIUM NIT. (URANIUM NITRATE)
Useful in the treatment of sugar diabetes
and also diabetes insipidus. Reduces
thirst and urine output.

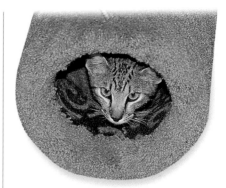

*Nervous and fearful
behavior is calmed by the
remedy Phosphorus.*

URTICA (STINGING NETTLE)
Relieves irritating and burning skin
conditions; rashes, allergies, eczema.
Promotes flow of milk, and of urine.

USTILLAGO (CORN SMUT)
A male and female hormonal balancing
remedy. Helps reduces unwanted male
behavior.

VERATRUM ALB. (WHITE HELLEBORE)
A remedy for collapse and diarrhea.
Patient is cold, with a weak pulse.

ZINC (ZINC)
For anemia, conjunctivitis with lack of
tear production, and epileptic patients
with a sensitivity to noise.

*When choosing a remedy remember to
assess the whole constitution, not only
the physical symptoms.*

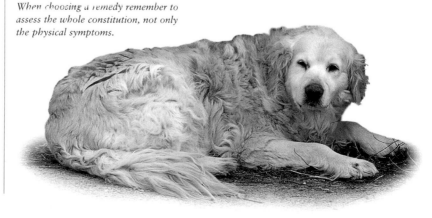

Crystals and Gems

Modern life would fall apart without crystals. Silicon chips are essentially thin slices of quartz crystals and we all know that there are chips in everything these days. Computers, cars, and communications are all dependent on crystals in the form of chips. Why? Because quartz crystals have a unique ability to amplify, focus, transform, and transfer energy.

This ability has another, older use – to heal. Crystal healing is energy medicine. It amplifies and directs energy into diseased parts of the body to harmonize and heal the imbalanced energy of the damaged area. By placing crystals on or close to pets that are ill, remarkable healing effects can often be induced. Crystals can be sewn into collars, put in halters, or simply placed next to resting animals.

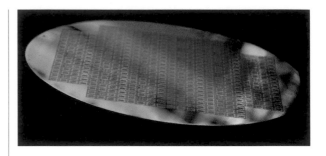

This silicon chip is made from millions of layers of quartz.

CRYSTAL ENERGY

Crystals amplify the whole energy field of the body, but if placed at a particular point in the body will focus energy more strongly in that area. So a crystal worn on the neck will stimulate the thyroid gland and be particularly useful for respiratory problems such as sore throat and sinus congestion. Crystals placed near the solar plexus will help abdominal problems.

As well as possessing a store of energy that is a natural healing and harmonizing force, crystals are often used by healers to help amplify and focus their own healing energy. You can use this amplifying effect of crystals when your pet is ill. Hold a crystal over the area of the body that needs healing, and then clear your mind and think positive thoughts. Imagine the healing process, and the problem dissolving.

You can't overdose with crystals; they can be left in place for long periods of time, but as well as accepting positive energy, crystals can also pick up negative energy. For this

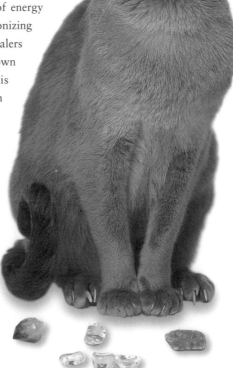

reason, crystals should always be cleansed before use. Wash with cool water (preferably mineral or filtered water) and brush any dirt out if necessary, then let dry in the open air. Finally, hold the crystal and visualize positive energy flowing in – this will also help personalize it.

One hi-tech way of using crystals is electrocrystal therapy. In this technique, an electric charge of variable frequency is passed through a mixture of different types of quartz crystals in a saline solution, in a sealed tube. By varying the frequency, the energy of particular crystals can be amplified, so increasing the healing effect enormously. The tube is then placed on the part of the body that corresponds with the specific healing effect of the crystal being energized. Gemstones have similar healing effects to crystals and both are suitable for all pets.

Crystals and gems are available from specialist shops and by mail order. There is not enough room here to detail the wide range of crystals and gems, but the following condensed list includes the most useful ones.

Crystals have a remarkable healing effect and can cure all types of physical and mental ills.

CRYSTALS AND THEIR QUALITIES

AGATE
Available in many colors and types; all improve vitality and strength, and neutralize anger and resentful feelings. Brown agate is used for fevers, epilepsy, and fluid retention.

AMBER
Strengthening and detoxifying. Used to relieve stomach pains and toothache. Promotes good liver and kidney functions.

AMETHYST
A strong healing crystal. Neutralizes harmful radiation. Good for eye disease including cataracts. Increases energy, but also aids restful sleep.

AVENTURINE
A balancing stone. Green Aventurine heals the body, Blue Aventurine heals mental problems, and Peach Aventurine heals emotional traumas.

BERYL
Enhances willpower and strength of mind. Useful for pets during long-term illness, or cancer. Green Beryl treats eye disease; Yellow Beryl treats jaundice.

BLUE LACE AGATE
A powerful anti-arthritic remedy; relieves symptoms of stiffness and pain. Also for repeated throat infections.

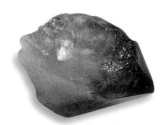
Amethyst

CARNELION (BLOODSTONE)
As its name suggests, used for persistent hemorrhage, reddened skin, and any blood disorder.

CELESTITE
Brings out the softer side of snappy or aggressive animals. Fosters the human-animal bond. It is said to increase the telepathic powers of pets!

CHALCEDONY
A nourishing, nurturing stone. Increases stamina and physical energy. Reduces temperature in fevers.

CHRYSOPRASE
Stimulates willpower in pets that seem to be giving in to severe illnesses. Protects against new or re-infections.

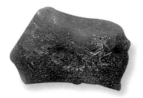
Amber

CITRINE
Generally used to promote well-being in pets that seem depressed or ill at ease.

CLEAR QUARTZ
Cleanses and detoxifies, and is a general healer for all conditions.

GLACIATED COPPER
Formed into unusual shapes by ice glaciers, copper stone is an effective remedy for stiff and swollen joints, back problems and arthritis.

DIAMOND
For eyes, ear, and nose disease. Also facial paralysis, coughs, and bronchitis and other lung diseases. Tonsillitis and similar throat conditions.

FUCHSITE
A soft pale green stone, used for skin complaints, particularly allergies, eczema, and skin infections.

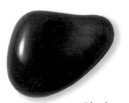
Blue lace agate

GALENA
A grounding stone for pets that seem to be "up in the clouds" – they don't respond to commands and sometimes seem in a trance.

GARNET
Good for skin diseases, especially wet eczema, or for skin with recurring infections that have not responded to other treatment.

HAEMATITE
Good for hemorrhage, especially from lungs or uterus. Bloodshot eyes. Also protects against sunstroke.

JADE (CHINESE)
Treats kidney problems, especially if fluid retention is present. Also for eye problems, heart weakness, and as an aid to easy delivery for pregnant pets.

JET
A remedy for toothache, pains in the head, glandular swellings, and epilepsy.

KYANITE
Stimulates the mental abilities of dull, lethargic pets. Good to restore confidence and abilities of pets from rescue centers.

LABRADORITE
Promotes healing in pets during long illnesses, when they seem to be losing willpower.

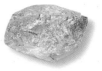
Diamond

LAPIS LAZULI

A pain-relieving remedy – for pains anywhere in the body, but particularly in the head, eyes, or ears. Also used to prevent miscarriage in pets prone to spontaneous abortion.

LODESTONE (MAGNETITE)

Used to counteract negative energies in or around the home, such as electricity pylons, nearby power stations, radio and television transmitters – or even noisy neighbors or traffic fumes. Place one lodestone in each of the four corners of the home.

MOONSTONE

Treats female hormone imbalances, uterine infections, vaginal discharges. A general anti-inflammatory remedy.

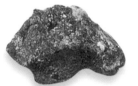

Lapis lazuli

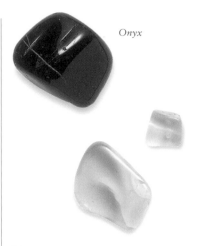

Onyx

Moonstone

OBSIDIAN

Also known as Apache Tears. Used for emotional traumas such as depression and lack of appetite after the loss of a companion (animal or human).

ONYX

Treats stomach upsets with excess acidity, burning sensations in general, glandular swellings, and brain disorders such as meningitis.

OPAL

Used for centuries for eye diseases of all kinds. Also helps stabilize nervous and hysterical animals.

PEARL

For respiratory diseases – asthma, bronchitis, and coughing up mucus. Also for kidney disease and chronic arthritic conditions.

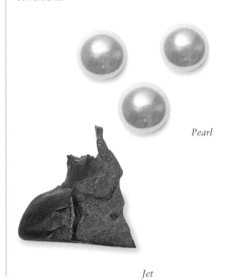

Pearl

Jet

Cystal and gem therapy can revitalize a pet that has become dull and lethargic.

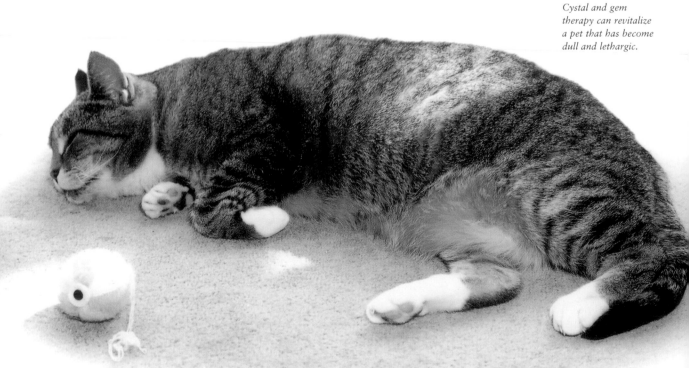

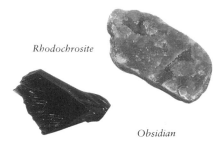

Rhodochrosite

Obsidian

PREHENITE
Another protective stone. Useful to protect the patient against side-effects of conventional drugs, especially radiotherapy and chemotherapy.

RHODOCHROSITE
Helpful for pets that are resentful or irritable in new situations; move of home or new arrival – baby or other pet.

RHODONITE
A training aid for pets that can't seem to see the point of instructions and keep forgetting what to do.

ROSE QUARTZ
For aggression and for over-dominant pets, to enable them to live in harmony with animal and human companions.

RUBY
A remedy for disorders of the blood – anemia, leukemia, hemorrhage. Used at any time of weakness, debility, lethargy. For collapse with a weak pulse and cold body.

SAPPHIRE
Mainly for nervous system disease, neuritis, nerve pain from slipped discs and trapped nerves. Also for depression and confused mental states, for instance in senile pets.

SARDONYX
For young pets, helps bodily – and mental – development. Also gives confidence to pets at times of change in life – new home, new owner.

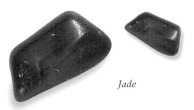

Jade

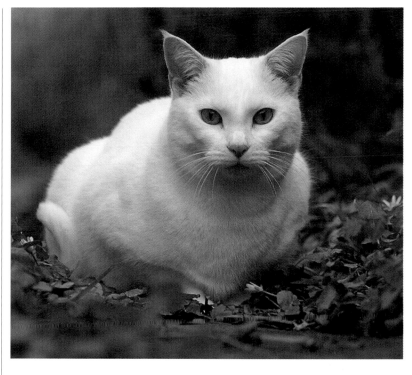

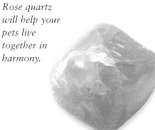

Rose quartz will help your pets live together in harmony.

SODALITE
For metabolic imbalances, such as thyroid dysfunction, pancreatic problems, or adrenal gland disease. Generally calming and soothing.

STIBNITE
For pets that can never keep still and concentrate, always wanting to be up and doing something, never playing with one toy for long.

SUGULITE
Strengthens body's healing powers when under stress, useful in the treatment of cancer and other serious illnesses.

TOPAZ
Detoxifying, strengthening, and restorative – sometimes described as the antidote to modern life. Particularly

ABOVE *Protect your pet from airborne pollutants and chemicals with turquoise.*

useful at times of severe air pollution, for stress, and to neutralize sources of electromagnetic radiation. Specific for sore throats, loss of voice, sore eyes, itchy skin, and insect stings and bites.

TOURMALINE
A remedy to help fears and phobias – especially fear of thunder, fireworks, or loud noises in general; and fears of meeting strangers (animal or human). Generally calming and soothing.

TURQUOISE
Strong healer – for eye disease, urinary problems, insect and snake bites. Also a protector against pollutants, especially airborne chemicals.

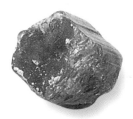

Tourmaline

Massage and Manipulation

All the therapies that use methods of massage and manipulation, such as osteopathy, chiropractic, and physiotherapy, involve the use of physical techniques and touch on the body. In its simplest form, such physical therapy is rubbing, stroking, adjusting, and manipulating, but it can, in terms of physiotherapy, include physical techniques such as the use of ultrasound, electrical and magnetic stimulation, heat and cold, stretching and compression.

Stroking a pet is enjoyable for both owner and pet as a pleasurable experience, but physical therapy takes us beyond this into the realms of treatment of illness and disease. From simple massage techniques that can be used at home, to the more sophisticated techniques of osteopathy, chiropractic, and physiotherapy – which can be used only by trained professionals – massage and manipulation is an effective, calming, natural therapy.

Kirlian photograph showing the heatspots created when applying massage strokes.

MASSAGE

Stroking your pet thoroughly, all over, is very effective. It gives your animal a soothing sensation; this will decrease tension, relax muscles, and tone the skin. At the same time, it gives the opportunity for you to feel for any lumps,

Stroking pets is enjoyable for both pet and owner.

bumps, warts, or other kinds of growths in the skin and lets you check for any signs of pain and discomfort in the body. While massaging you can also look for any signs of dandruff, fleas, ticks or other parasites, or any rashes or infections in the skin. Stroking and massage is therefore both therapeutic and potentially diagnostic, giving opportunity to identify early signs of disease in the area being stroked.

As a therapy there are several basic massage techniques. These are: effleurage – using the open palm and fingers to stroke slowly and lightly along the body, either along the back, or from hip to foot; fingertip – hold three fingers together and move the skin in a small circular motion over the underlying muscle; acupressure – apply pressure with thumb or finger to sensitive points (these points are often, but not always, points on the acupuncture meridian); petrissage – rolling the skin between finger and thumb and kneading it (over ligaments, tendons, and muscles, this can be done quite deeply to massage the muscle beneath the skin); and friction – fast, stroking massage with the balls of several fingers, smoothly but quickly applied. Always retain one hand on the body.

Specialist forms of massage include: aromatherapy massage – using essential oils to enhance the healing effect of the physical massage; Reiki – a form of laying-on of hands (spiritual healing), which uses specific energy centers in the body; and Tellington T-touch – this is a method of massage developed by Linda Tellington-Jones based on the Feldenkrais method, a human massage and movement therapy. The Tellington T-touch is a system of gentle, repeated massaging movements, which generate specific behavior patterns in the patient. This massage is especially beneficial for pets suffering from anxiety, especially following injuries or surgery. There are many variations on a theme, but most T-touch massage involves using small circular massaging movements, repeated regularly for 15 minutes at a time.

CHIROPRACTIC AND OSTEOPATHY

These more manipulative therapies involve concentrating mainly on the spine as the source of a great deal of physical disease in all species. Neither should be attempted at home; both therapies must be performed on any pet by a qualified professional only. A number of sessions may be required for a long-term problem such as arthritis but for a short-term problem, such as a pulled muscle, a single session may be sufficient to solve the problem.

Chiropractic involves small adjustments to the spinal column by applying firm but gentle pressure at points along the spine. Chiropractic states that there is a strong relationship between the physical state of the spinal column and that of the nervous system, and that the spinal column is the pivot of the whole skeleton. If the spine can successfully be adjusted and malformations put right or minimized by careful applications of chiropractic techniques, then the whole body, especially the nervous system, will become more healthy and some diseases at least will be eliminated from the body.

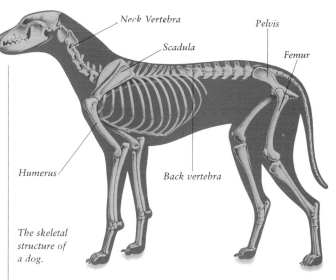

The skeletal structure of a dog.

Neck Vertebra
Scadula
Pelvis
Femur
Humerus
Back vertebra

Osteopathy involves more physical manipulation. It can occasionally look quite violent, if a spine is to be stretched, for instance. Osteopathy may also overlap physiotherapy in including stretching, and the use of hot and cold compresses as part of the session.

MASSAGE

•Always start massage sessions with a few gentle strokes and then build up the strength and direction of the stroke into one of the basic massage techniques.

•Always massage with the lie of the fur on the skin, not against it.

•Massage improves circulation to damaged areas of tissue, helping to remove excess fluid, toxins, and poisons. It also stimulates the release of natural painkillers by the body.

•Massage should be carried out regularly – once or twice a week on healthy animals – to obtain maximum benefit as a diagnostic method to detect early disease, and to act as a soothing, toning procedure.

•Give a daily massage to animals with mental or emotional problems, or with

Massage strokes should always follow the direction of fur growth.

physical conditions such as pulled muscles or sprained tendons or ligaments.

• Massage is suitable for most pets. Even reptiles appreciate a stroking massage once you get to know them well.

• Therapeutic massage for more serious forms of disease should be carried out only by a trained professional.

• Massage and manipulation should always be included as part of a natural approach to the treatment of injuries, particularly in the healing of joint, muscle, ligament, tendon, and nerve damage.

PHYSIOTHERAPY

Physiotherapy involves the use of specific physical techniques in the treatment of disease. These include:

ELECTRICAL

Modern electrical stimulators emit a safe, smooth output that is used to give pain relief, stimulate blood and lymph circulation, and help develop weak or damaged muscles. The best known use of electric therapy is TENS – Transcutaneous Electrical Nerve Stimulator. Electrical physiotherapy may be used on most pets (except fish), size being the only limiting factor.

Modern electrical stimulators can be safely used on most pets to give pain relief, stimulate circulation, and to develop and relieve weak or damaged muscles.

ULTRASOUND

Ultrasound involves the use of ultra high-frequency sound waves to increase the temperature of body tissues. This speeds healing of ligaments and tendons and also reduces scarring. Ultrasound combined with physical stretching exercise is profoundly effective in treating sprains, strains, joint disease, and muscle injuries. Typically, a five-minute ultrasound session may be given once a week for four weeks, with gentle stretching exercises between sessions, in the treatment of severe sprains.

Ultrasound should not be used just after exercise, and overuse will cause overheating of tissues. Only a trained physiotherapist should administer ultrasound. It is suitable for most pets (except fish), although very small pets can be difficult to treat.

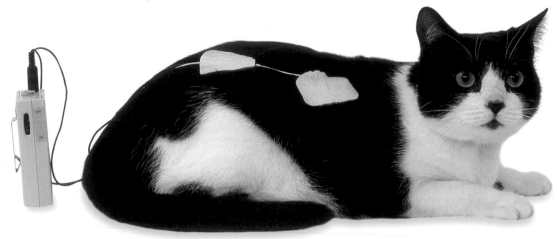

HEAT, COLD, AND COMPRESSION

HEAT

Infra-red lamps, warm water baths, electric heating pads, and hot packs all provide local heat to damaged tissue. These heat superficially, and do not provide the deeper heat penetration of ultrasound. Local heat stimulation is useful in increasing circulation, and in pain relief. Rubbing a painful spot after an injury is giving both massage and local heat therapy from the friction of the rubbing. More specific heat applications, such as an infra-red lamp, give longer lasting relief from soreness and pain, and increase the healing rate after injuries. Heat application should be used only under the direction of a trained physiotherapist. It is suitable for most pets (except fish), but extreme care must be taken in the case of smaller pets below the size of cats.

Small animals can be treated with heat stimulation by a physiotherapist.

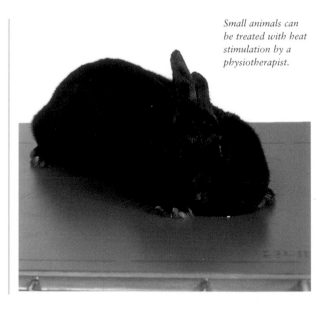

COLD AND COMPRESSION

Ice is a very effective physical therapy. A ten-minute application of an ice pack can reduce blood flow to the treated area by 70 percent. The effect of cold is enhanced by applying pressure at the same time. Pressure will naturally limit blood flow to the affected area. Gel ice packs, used in insulated picnic boxes and available from supermarkets, are very convenient to use. A plastic cup filled with water and then frozen provides an ideal alternative. A plastic bag full of ice cubes can also be used. In emergencies, a bag of frozen peas will do perfectly well.

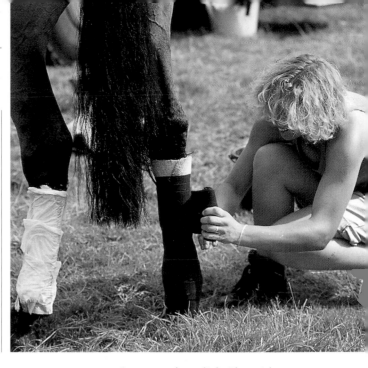

Pressure can be applied with special compression wraps and bandages.

• Pressure can be applied using simple pressure from the hands or by using compression wraps and bandages. It should be used for short periods only – not more than 15 minutes at a time.
• Hosing with cold water provides only a minimal cooling effect; ice packs are much more effective.
• Cold and compression act as a local anesthetic, and give good pain relief after an injury.
• Regular use of cold and compression must be under the direction of a trained physiotherapist.
• Cold and compression therapy are suitable for all but the smallest pets.

In an emergency, a bag of frozen peas will serve very well as an ice pack.

• Alternate hot and cold compresses are used by physiotherapists for some conditions.

STRETCHING

Stretching exercises strengthen weakened and damaged muscles and joints, and improve flexibility. Stretching is the best-known treatment given by physiotherapists. A combination of heat followed by stretching is often used. When an animal is recovering from injury, a trained physiotherapist may devise a routine of carefully assessed movements to stretch and strengthen the affected joints and muscles and improve mobility.

Knowing which kind of stretching to use, for how long, and how frequently, needs training and expertise. Never begin stretching exercises on your pet without the advice and supervision of a trained physiotherapist. Avoid manual stretching when acute inflammation is present, or if the patient finds it painful. Over-stretching can damage joints and muscles.

LASERS

The therapeutic use of lasers is discussed in more detail on page 26. Here are some points to remember:
• Laser therapy is especially effective in treating ulcers, and non-healing wounds and burns, deep cuts, as well as scar tissue.
• Laser light machines are now, in most cases, produced in small, portable forms, including a pen laser (often used for small cuts or bruises).
• Light therapy is suitable for all pets, except fish.
• A low-output, battery-operated, pocket-sized laser pen is safe for home use for first aid treatment – wounds, scratches, inflamed ears – but not as a replacement for veterinary treatment. Advice in the use of a laser pen must be obtained from a skilled practitioner before use.

EMERGENCY

After an injury, an ice pack and compression should be applied to the affected area as soon as possible to give pain relief and reduce hemorrhage and bruising.
Heat should not be used until three days after an injury, to avoid aggravating any swelling and bleeding. But after three days heat therapy will improve blood supply to the damaged area and bring further relief, removing toxins, and increasing the rate of healing.

Nutritional Therapy

Food as medicine is a concept dating back to the ancient Greeks. A wide variety of nutrients can be used to heal damaged tissue, reduce inflammation in joints, strengthen the immune system, improve energy, and treat diseases such as cancer.

To obtain this healing effect, such nutrients are often given in far higher doses than would normally be found in natural food sources. They are therefore being used as therapeutic medicines rather than simply as nutrients, hence the term nutritional therapy.

Among the massive range of possible nutritional therapeutic agents, the most useful and effective in animals include vitamins, minerals, amino acids, essential fatty acids, enzymes, probiotics, and, of course, fruit and vegetables.

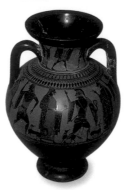

The understanding of food as medicine dates back to the ancient Greeks.

VITAMINS

VITAMIN C

High doses of vitamin C will help to treat allergies, infections, stress, cancer, liver disease, gum disease, and arthritis, and will speed up the healing of wounds. The body does not store the vitamin so it is not possible to overdose on it.

• It is especially required by guinea pigs to prevent scurvy and to treat lung infections such as pneumonia.

• Dose rates of up to 2 g for a large dog, or 100 mg daily for a guinea pig are typical.

VITAMIN E

Vitamin E is an antioxidant and is most effective in the treatment of heart disease, cataracts, skin disease, and nerve damage. CDRM (see page 120) in large dogs is treated with large doses of vitamin E (2000 iu daily).

VITAMIN A

Vitamin A is a useful treatment for skin diseases and as an immune system booster. It also protects against damage caused by pollutants and carcinogens and is useful in treating cataracts and other eye diseases. It can be toxic in high doses – obtain veterinary advice if using it as a nutritional therapy.

• Abnormal eggs in birds (soft- or rough-shelled or yolkless) can be treated with a combination of calcium and vitamins D and A.

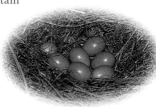

Abnormal shells are caused by vitamin and mineral deficiency.

VITAMIN B COMPLEX

This is useful for dealing with stress, allergies, and infections and is another immune system booster.

Often given in the form of Brewer's yeast – a key product of the brewing industry – which is rich in B-complex vitamins.

• Tortoises not eating after coming out of hibernation are treated with B-complex vitamins to improve appetite and boost the immune system.

• Too much can cause diarrhea in birds.

BIOTIN

This is one of the B-complex group, initially called vitamin H. Biotin improves and strengthens the condition of nails and feet pads. It also helps prevent nail bed infection. It is often used in horses to help with hoof abnormalities, and reduces flaking and cracking of nails in all animals.

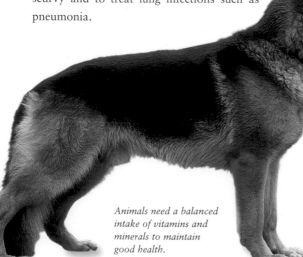

Animals need a balanced intake of vitamins and minerals to maintain good health.

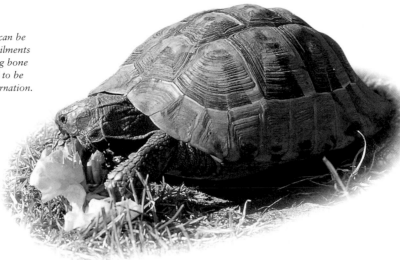

Nutritional therapy can be used to treat many ailments in tortoises, including bone disease and the need to be revitalized after hibernation.

MINERALS

ZINC

Treats skin disease where there is flaking, dandruff, and itchiness of the skin, especially where mange mites or allergies are present.

CALCIUM

This can treat various skeletal problems. In addition, egg problems, such as egg-binding or soft-shelled eggs, and nutritional osteodystrophy (bone disease) in tortoises and lizards are helped with extra calcium, given with the correct balance of phosphorus. This is usually available as a combined supplement in tablet from.

IODINE

This can help treat thyroid imbalances. It is often given in the form of kelp, a seaweed rich in iodine and other vitamins and minerals.

• Budgerigars may suffer from a thyroid imbalance, which makes them emit a high pitched "squeaky door" sound; this can be treated with iodine.

Supplementary calcium can be used to treat bone disease in reptiles.

AMINO ACIDS

These are the building blocks of protein and have many uses in the body. The most common are:

• L-Carnitine – useful in the treatment of heart disease, especially endocardiosis, congestive heart failure, and dilated cardiomyopathy.

• Glutamine – an ideal treatment for inflammatory bowel disease. It minimizes the loss of muscle mass that occurs at times of stress, injury, and excessive exercise.

• Dimethylglycine – this improves stamina and is especially effective as an immune system booster. It particularly helps animals with chronic viral infections, such as feline leukemia and the feline immunodeficiency virus. It also has an anti-inflammatory effect.

• Taurine – this is an essential component of the diet of cats, since they cannot manufacture it themselves. Lack of taurine causes eye disease. A deficiency can also leads to heart damage.

Doses of 500 mg to 1000 mg will help treat heart conditions such as dilated cardiomyopathy.

ESSENTIAL FATTY ACIDS (EFAS)

EFAS are commonly used in the treatment of skin disease in dogs and cats. They reduce the shedding of hair, minimize dandruff and flaky skin, relieve dryness and greasiness of skin, treat allergic problems, and help in the treatment of arthritis, cancer, and kidney disorders. They are found in large amounts in evening primrose oil, borage oil, and blackcurrant seed oil, and also in fish oils – cod, halibut, and salmon. A combination of plant and fish oils often gives best results in treatment.

Evening primrose

COENZYME Q10

This is an enzyme naturally produced in mammals, which controls the uptake and use of oxygen by body cells. Production of coenzyme Q10 decreases with age, so older animals will often benefit from a Q10 supplement. It is used as a treatment for two major conditions – heart disorders and gum and mouth disease. Dramatic improvement is often seen within two weeks of starting coenzyme Q10 treatment.

• Gingivitis (gum inflammation) in dogs and cats responds well to this supplement.

PROANTHOCYANIDIN COMPLEX

Also known as bioflavinoids and pycnogenols, proanthocyanidins are compounds found in plants. They are natural antioxidants, and are useful as immune system boosters in anti-allergic therapy, and as anticancer treatment. They are found in many fruits and seeds, ranging from pine bark to grape seed. Vitamin C with added bioflavinoids is a potent remedy to boost the immune system, especially after illness.

PERNA MUSSEL

Perna, or green-lipped, mussels are raised commercially in New Zealand. For over 20 years, perna mussel extract has been used for both humans and animals as an anti-inflammatory agent in the treatment of arthritis. The main active ingredients are GAGs (glycosaminoglycans, see below).

Grape seed is a natural antioxident.

• Small pets can benefit – in one study 50 percent of mice with stiffness and arthritis responded well to dosing.

• Perna seems to slow the aging process – skin remains more elastic and coat condition improves, and joint stiffness seems less noticeable.

GLYCOSAMINOGLYCANS (GAGs)

These are a group of compounds that provide the structure and flexibility for cartilage and connective tissue. Combined with proteins, they form the complete tissue. They are large molecules, made up of many small components called glucosamines. The most important types are chondroitin sulphate and hyaluronic acid.

• Supplementing with GAGs will help to rebuild the worn cartilage of osteoarthritis, to hinder deterioration in joints and to renew damaged tissue.

• GAGs have a natural anti-inflammatory effect, and

Shark cartilage has many medicinal uses.

improve the viscosity (stickiness) of joint fluid – in other words, improve the lubrication.

• GAGs are used in the treatment of many cartilage and spinal disc degenerative diseases, such as arthritis, hip dysplasia, spondylitis, and osteochronditis.

• Glucosamines, the building blocks of GAGs, can be administered in a similar way as a treatment for arthritis. Glucasomines are also found in the lining of the bowel, and can be used as part of a treatment regime for inflammatory bowel allergies and recurrent colitis. Gastroentrinal illness can be responsive to glucosamine treatment.

PROBIOTICS

Probiotics are bacteria that are naturally present in the digestive tract, and have a beneficial function in supplying nutrients to the body, helping digestive processes, and using

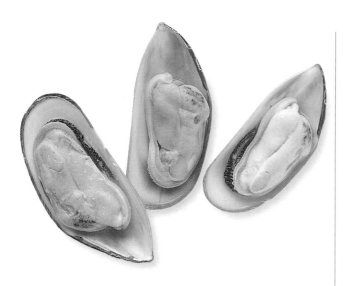

Extracts from green-lipped or Perna mussels are used in the treatment of arthritis.

food more efficiently. Using these bacteria as treatment will therefore help with a variety of digestive disorders. The most commonly used probiotics are lactobacilli.

• Antibiotics destroy both harmful and beneficial bacteria in the gut. Always give probiotics after a course of antibiotics. This will reduce the likelihood of bowel disturbance, and speed return of normal bowel flora.

• Probiotics are available as bacteria-rich powders or capsules, and occur in large numbers in live, plain yogurt. Commercially-sold, sweetened, flavored, and pasteurized yogurts contain few, if any bacteria.

• Apart from using probiotics after antibiotics, it is also important to treat pets suffering from any condition that can upset or imbalance the digestive tract – stress, fevers, or injuries to the abdomen. Stresses that can adversely affect the gastrointestinal balance include sudden change of diet, malnutrition, weaning, traveling long distances, and poor housing.

• Probiotics do not have long shelf lives, and should be refrigerated and used immediately.

• For animals with long-term digestive problems, probiotics can be given over an extended period of time. However, in most cases they are used for two to three weeks at a time. This is in cases following antibiotic use or at times of stress or infections.

• Probiotics are suitable for all mammals, but are not usually effective in fish, reptiles, birds, or chelonians (tortoises and terrapins).

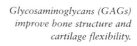

Glycosaminoglycans (GAGs) improve bone structure and cartilage flexibility.

CARTILAGE PRODUCTS

Cartilage from both sharks and cattle contain high levels of natural anti-inflammatory agents and anticancer components. Both shark and bovine cartilage are effective against arthritis, disc and other spinal problems, and is beneficial in the treatment of cardiovascular problems and immune system disease.

The anti-inflammatory agents are mainly a group of naturally occurring substances called glycosaminoglycans (GAGs). These are part of the structure that gives cartilage and connective tissue its resilience, strength, and flexibility. (For more information on GAGs, see page 62). Apart from being an excellent natural source of GAGs, both shark and bovine cartilage contain natural anticancer agents that reduce the growth of new blood vessels in and

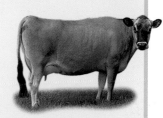

Bovine cartilage is an effective anti-inflammatory and anticancer agent.

around tumors. By reducing the blood supply, the tumor is effectively starved and may shrink or stop growing.

There are many concerns about the use of shark cartilage. Although it is often stated that sharks are not killed purely for their cartilage, it is difficult to prove this on balance. Thus, it is preferable to use other cartilage products.

FRUIT AND VEGETABLES

Fruits and vegetables are a good source of natural medicines. Some pets will eat fruit and vegetables happily and naturally; others may have to be persuaded. In small amounts, they are safe for all pets, except fish and some totally carnivorous species, such as carnivorous snakes. However, stop giving such foods if diarrhea or other digestive problems occur.

Fruits and vegetables should always be fresh and, ideally, organic. Wash non-organic thoroughly.

FRUIT

• Apples improve digestion generally, and relieve constipation. Do not feed pips.

• Apricots are good for respiratory infections. Laetrile, extracted from apricot kernels, has been used successfully to treat cancer.

• Do not feed apricot stones – they contain a substance that can be broken down in the digestive tract to form prussic acid.

• Bananas contain high levels of potassium, which is useful to help prevent strokes or reduce the likelihood of recurrence of strokes.

• Cider vinegar is a natural antiseptic. Add 1 teaspoon per 1¼ pints (600 ml) of drinking water to help treat arthritis, cystitis, and bowel infections.

• Cranberries are an anticystitis remedy. Pets prone to cystitis should be given cranberry juice daily; you can dilute it in filtered water to encourage consumption.

• Cranberry drinks and sauces usually contain sugars and are not recommended.

• Figs help combat constipation, and are also good for pets that suffer repeated abscesses.

• Grapes are a cleansing agent and detoxifier – good for liver problems.

• Kiwi fruit are used for circulatory and digestive disorders; and because of its vitamin C content, it is a good supplement to an anticancer treatment regime.

• Pineapple juice is ideal for soothing sore throats. It contains an enzyme that helps reduce bruising.

• Strawberry juice rubbed on the teeth helps reduce build-up of tartar and plaque. Strawberries are beneficial when kidney stones are present.

VEGETABLES

• Asparagus is a natural mild diuretic, and will help in treating heart disease, and some kidney and liver disorders.

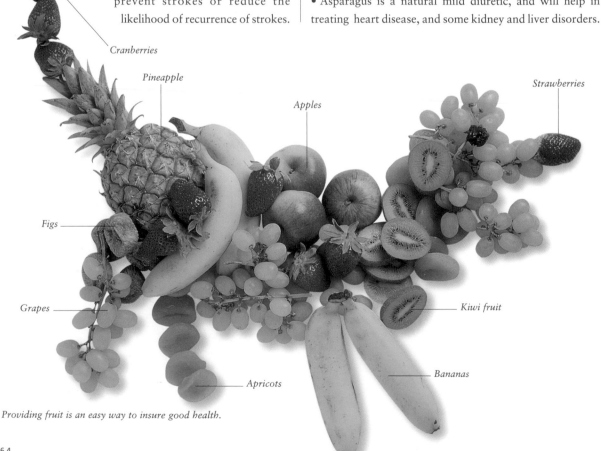

Cranberries

Pineapple

Apples

Strawberries

Figs

Grapes

Kiwi fruit

Apricots

Bananas

Providing fruit is an easy way to insure good health.

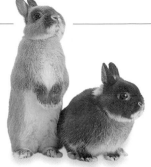

Rabbits can be fed a wide variety of fresh fruit and vegetables. Non-organic produce should be carefully washed.

• Beet is good for bladder infections, and also liver disease. Beet juice is a purifier and can help in the treatment of eczema.

• Broccoli is high in levels of sulfurophanes, which are natural anticancer agents, and so should be added to the diet of pets with cancer.

• Do not feed broccoli to pets with underactive thyroids.

• Cabbage juice is helpful in the treatment of mouth ulcers and gastric (stomach) ulcers.

• Like broccoli, cabbage contains sulfurophane and should not be given to pets with underactive thyroids.

• Carrots are well known for their use in improving eyesight (carrots can help to prevent cataract formation), and they are also a mild diuretic and can help to treat cystitis.

• Celery seeds are a natural anti-arthritic agent often given with willow bark as a treatment for arthritis. Do not give to pregnant pets.

• Cucumber juice is a good cystitis treatment, and is also helpful in cases of eczema.

• Lettuce contains natural calming agents, both for mental anxiety and nervousness and for all physical conditions such as irritable bowel syndrome.

• Onion in small amounts is anti-infective, and is particularly good for respiratory infection.

• Onions in large amounts are poisonous – give for a few days at a time only.

• Pumpkin seeds are used to treat prostate disease, as part of an anticancer diet, and when ground into a powder can be administered to help prevent worm infestation.

• Radishes are useful as antibacterial and antifungal agents. They are also beneficial for flatulence and bloating of the lower intestines.

• Radishes should not be given to pets with gastric inflammation or ulcers.

• Corn has fine silk hairs which can be gathered and made into an infusion that is a natural diuretic. Cornsilk infusion also soothes the stomach when gastritis is present.

• Watercress is a useful respiratory remedy for catarrh and bronchitis. Also used for eczema, general debility, and anemia.

• Do not give watercress to pets suffering from cystitis.

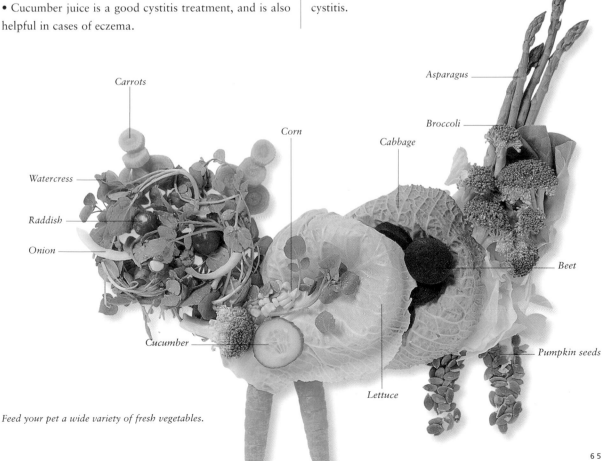

Carrots

Corn

Asparagus

Broccoli

Cabbage

Watercress

Raddish

Onion

Beet

Cucumber

Pumpkin seeds

Lettuce

Feed your pet a wide variety of fresh vegetables.

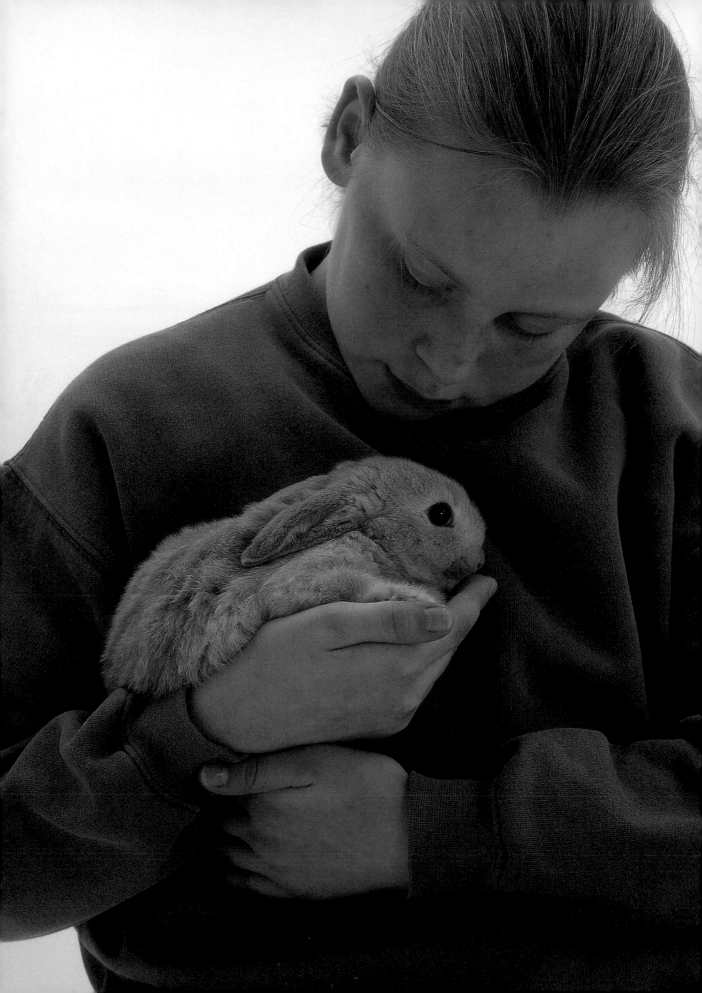

Part III

Common Ailments

We are all so used to visiting our doctor for treatment when we feel unwell, or taking our pet to the veterinarian when illness strikes, that taking responsibility for our own health is a big step; taking responsibility for our pet's health is an even bigger issue. Pets are so dependent on us – for their food, water, and safety, as well as their health – that it seems natural for us to let the experts help with maintaining our pets' health; and of course, medical and veterinary services offer a great deal to us and our pets.

> ### THE BASIC RULES ABOUT USING NATURAL THERAPIES ARE:
>
> • If your pet is seriously ill (or you think it may be seriously ill), call your veterinary practice right away. It is safe to use natural medicines while you are awaiting veterinary attention.
>
> • If your pet has a minor ailment, begin treating with natural remedies, but call your veterinarian if the condition worsens rapidly, or there is no improvement in a few days.

COMPLEMENTARY MEDICINE

However, except in a few instances, they do not offer a true choice of treatments. In addition to conventional Western drug medicine and surgery, there is a vast array of safe, effective natural remedies available.

Treating ailments naturally lets you harness this huge reservoir of knowledge to the advantage of your pet. In the following pages, you will find descriptions of all the common small animal diseases. Each body system and its diseases are examined in turn. There are sections on viral, bacterial, and other microorganism diseases and chapters on topics from cancer to parasites. The mind is also taken into account, with pages on mental, emotional, and behavioral problems. In all cases, conditions and symptoms are explained, causes identified, and natural medicines are detailed.

Treating animals can be quite nerve-racking. Don't worry – all the remedies shown are safe to use with the instructions given. But always consult your veterinarian if in doubt. Let common sense be your guide; usually we know whether our pet is slightly unwell or needing rapid veterinary attention.

Observe your pet and handle it very frequently so that you can spot early signs if illness.

Throughout the treatment section there will be pointers highlighted to guide you as to whether to take your pet to the veterinarian immediately, or to use natural remedies first.

The previous chapters on the individual therapies have described what therapies can be used for pets, how to prepare the remedies, and how to administer them. When a remedy is mentioned as a treatment for a disease, refer back to these sections for information on how to prepare and administer the remedy, and what dose rate to use.

ESSENTIAL REMEDIES

It is a good idea to keep a store of natural medicines available. Be prepared, and have in store at least the top ten homeopathic remedies and a selection of herbs, crystals, essential oils, and flower and gem remedies. Arnica and Rescue Remedy are a must, but you will also need the back-up of a small selection of remedies to cope with common, minor ailments. It is also wise to have a first-aid kit, with bandages, to deal with wounds and other minor injuries.

Above all, take time to observe and check your pet regularly. Early signs of illness are always important. Learn how warm your pet normally feels, so that you detect any increase in temperature; check eyes and ears regularly for signs of discharge or soreness; notice how much your pet normally eats and drinks, so that any variation will be quickly obvious; run your hands over your pet's body daily to check for lumps and swellings or signs of discomfort. Basically, get to know what is normal, and you will rapidly detect the abnormal.

Now you are ready to deal with cuts and bruises, upset stomachs, cystitis, sore ears, itchy skin – the everyday complaints that can occasionally affect the fittest, healthiest pet. Read on – and learn how to heal your pet the natural way!

Abscess

CAUSES

Bacterial infection caused by:
- bites
- cuts
- wounds
- insect stings

SIGNS AND SYMPTOMS

- swelling
- pain
- discomfort
- may be reddened and hot to touch
- may discharge pus

An abscess is a swelling containing pus, which forms as a result of bacterial infection. An abscess can occur almost anywhere in the body, but most form under the skin, as a result of bites, cuts, wounds, or insect stings.

Symptoms are swelling, pain, and discomfort. The swelling and area around it may be reddened and hot to the touch. An abscess may come to a head and discharge pus.

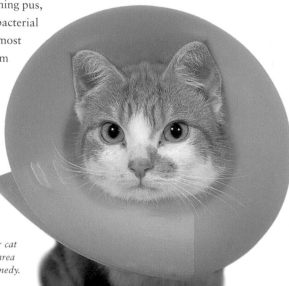

A lampshade collar will prevent your cat from repeatedly licking the affected area and removing any locally applied remedy.

DOS AND DON'TS

Don't burst an abscess.

Do encourage an abscess to come to a head by using a poultice or herbal draining ointment.

Do visit the veterinarian if your pet seems ill in general – high temperature, not eating, lethargy; the infection may have spread to the bloodstream and septicemia (blood poisoning) can result.

Do visit the veterinarian if multiple abscesses appear, or if an abscess continues to discharge.

Do look for reasons for repeated abscess formation – poor hygiene in caged pets, bullying by other animals, or impaired immune system.

REMEDIES

AROMATHERAPY
Apply **tea tree oil** (neat or diluted) three times daily.
Apply a compress of **camomile**, **lemon**, **lavender**, or **thyme** to bring the abscess out. Massage around the abscess with **galbanum**.

FLOWERS AND GEM REMEDIES
Crab apple or **camphor** as cleansing remedies.

HERBAL
Infusions of **red clove** or **thyme** are anti-infective. **Echinacea** boosts the immune system and fights infection. **Garlic** is antibacterial.

HOMEOPATHY
Apis mel. – for a hot, red, shiny abscess.
Graphites – for an interdigital abscess.
Hepar sulph – for a tender, painful abscess.
Lachesis – for a purple, discolored abscess, sensitive when touched.
Calc. sulph. – for the thick, cheesy pus of a discharging abscess.
Belladonna – for the early stage of an abscess: hot, throbbing, and painful.
All the above in acute dosage.

Silicea – for slow-forming abscesses that do not come to a head, or to help healing and minimize scarring in an old, healing abscess (chronic dosage).

CRYSTALS AND GEM ESSENCES
Amber for detoxifying when infection is active.
Fuchsite for infections in the skin.

NUTRITIONAL
Vitamin C boosts the immune system and fights infection.
Figs help prevent repeated abscesses.

Crab apple flower remedy is good for cleansing the system of toxins.

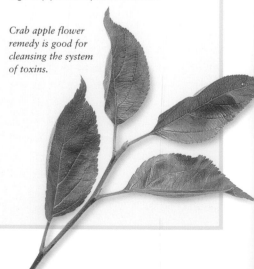

Alopecia

Alopecia is another name for baldness. Animals do not normally become bald naturally; although the fur or feathers may become thinner with age, large bald patches should not appear.

Many skin problems can cause fur loss, and it is important to find the underlying cause. Likely causes include hormonal imbalance (thyroid, adrenal, or male/female hormones), poor or imbalanced nutrition, skin infections, parasites (mites, ringworm, fleas), allergies, scars following burns or other injuries, immune system disease.

The symptoms of alopecia are fur or feather loss – this may be generalized, or may be in patches. If it is in patches that are bilaterally symmetrical (the same on either side) but is not itching, it is likely to be hormonal. If it is accompanied by itching and soreness, it is likely to be caused by parasites or allergies.

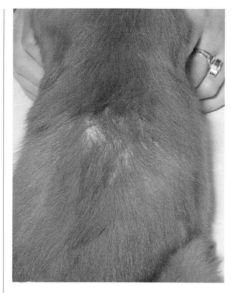

Loss of hair, fur, or feathers usually has an underlying cause.

There is no magic cure for baldness, but natural remedies can usually help to stimulate fur growth.

CAUSES

- hormonal imbalance
- poor nutrition
- skin infection
- parasites
- allergies
- scars
- immune system disease

SIGNS AND SYMPTOMS

- fur or feather loss may be accompanied by itching or soreness

REMEDIES

AROMATHERAPY
Many essential oils help promote new hair growth: **Angelica root**, **West Indian bay**, **elemi**, **grapefruit**, **juniper**, **ylang ylang**, **rosemary**, **lavender**, **thyme**.

Ginkgo stimulates hair growth and has a tonic affect on the entire circulation.

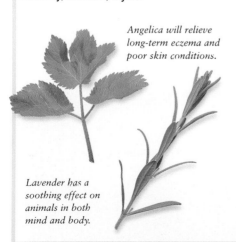

Angelica will relieve long-term eczema and poor skin conditions.

Lavender has a soothing effect on animals in both mind and body.

HERBAL
Dandelion, **ginkgo** and especially **kelp** all help.

CRYSTALS AND GEM ESSENCES
Garnet.

HOMEOPATHY
Thallium helps as a hair restorer.
Arsenicum album for hair loss accompanied by itching and dandruff.

NUTRITIONAL
Vitamin E and **biotin** both help with poor skin conditions.
Essential fatty acids are useful for alopecia with dry skin, dandruff, and itchiness.

DOS AND DON'TS

Don't ignore alopecia. The underlying cause could be serious – for instance, male animals with testicular cancer may develop alopecia.

Don't expect quick results. Hair often grows slowly – give it time.

Eczema

CAUSES

- allergy (direct contact with breathed in allergens)
- bacterial infection

SIGNS AND SYMPTOMS

- sore, itchy, flaky skin

SYMPTOMS

- dry eczema – dry, flaky, itchy skin; hair loss; variable degrees of redness.

- wet eczema – moist, sticky skin, often with infection and purulent discharge.

- seborrhea – greasy, oily skin with scaling, and often an unpleasant smell.

- chronic eczema – slowly progressing eczema, symptoms gradually worsening with time.

- acute eczema – sudden onset of severe, itchy skin.

The skin is the largest organ of the body – and the barrier between the outside and the body inside. It reflects external damage and internal changes. One of the commonest symptoms of this damage is eczema in its various forms.

Eczema essentially means inflamed skin. The term is more or less interchangeable with dermatitis. It is not a single condition, but a general term to describe an inflammatory reaction in the skin.

The symptoms can be classified in different ways. Indeed, eczema is frequently identified through description – see Symptoms panel, left.

Eczema can also be classified according to its cause, rather than descriptively. For instance, allergic eczema, pyoderma (eczema caused by bacterial infection), atopy (eczema caused by breathed-in allergens), contact dermatitis (eczema caused by direct contact with an allergen).

The interesting thing about all these different types of eczema is that the actual symptoms are in many cases identical. The skin has limited ways of reacting to the various causes of eczema. Essentially it becomes sore, itchy, and flaky to a lesser or greater extent, and that's it!

This is why skin problems can be so hard to diagnose, and even exhaustive tests may fail to find a definite cause. Treatment is equally difficult. A common saying is that

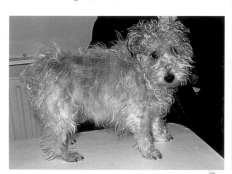

ABOVE *Dry eczema is recognized by its symptoms of dry and flaky skin, patchy hair loss, and localized itching.*

RIGHT *Roman camomile. This soothing oil treats rashes and dermatitis.*

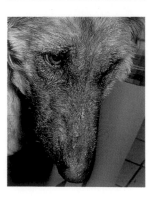

LEFT *Seborrhea results in patches of greasy, oily skin that flakes in scales and smells unpleasant.*

COLOR THERAPY
Yellow is the healing color for eczema, especially chronic dermatitis.

AROMATHERAPY
Many essential oils help when treating eczema.
Angelica root – for long-standing eczema and generally poor skin condition.
West Indian Bay – poor coat and scurfy, scaly skin.
Cajeput – for seborrhea: greasy, oily skin.
White camphor – chronic eczema.
Carrot seed – greasy skin, rashes.
Cedarwood – flaky and greasy skin, fungal infections, hair loss.
Roman camomile – dermatitis and rashes.
Galbanum – softens and heals damaged skin.
Juniper – all forms of eczema and hair loss.
Lavender – for all skin problems.
Eucalyptus – fungal and yeast skin conditions.
Orange – dull, dry, or greasy skin.
Patchouli – wet eczema; open sores, ringworm; scurfy, scaly skin.
Orange Petigrain – greasy skin and coat.
Rosemary – eczema, especially caused by parasites.
Clary sage – dandruff and flaking.
Sandalwood – dry, cracked skin.
Tagetes – thickened skin, fungal infections.
Ylang ylang – itchy skin, poor hair growth.

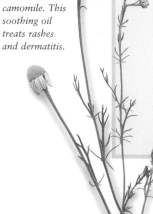

dermatologists do well because their patients never die from their condition – but nor do they get better!

This may not be quite true, but is an indication of how defensive eczema is to treatment. Conventional medicine is probably less effective at treating and controlling eczema than any other condition.

Natural medicines are extremely effective at coping with such skin conditions. However, the problem is in choosing from the multitude of potential remedies to use.

A selection of the most useful follows – but in most cases of eczema, particularly chronic, long-standing eczema, it is wise to get the advice of a veterinarian skilled in the use of natural remedies.

Because eczema may involve a combination of different causes, both internal and external, treating it is a complicated matter, needing much time and expertise.

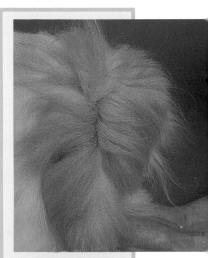

The condition known as stud tail affects cats only, usually males.

REMEDIES

FLOWER AND GEM REMEDIES
Cotton – for mange and other parasite causes of eczema.
Luffa – allergic eczema.

HERBAL
Aloe vera – used as a skin gel, this is a cooling, soothing agent ideal for the soreness and irritation caused by eczema. Also available as a spray, and can be taken by mouth. Ideal to grow in a conservatory for home use – just cut a leaf and squeeze the gel out.
Burdock – for eczema, especially when accompanied by liver disease.
Marigold – available as lotions and creams to relieve itching and soreness.
Echinacea – boosts the immune system and helps prevent or treat infected eczema (pyoderma).
Nettles – for allergic eczema where symptoms look like nettle rash.
Kelp – for poor skin and coat condition generally.

CRYSTAL AND GEM ESSENCES
Coral, **fuchsite**, and **garnet** all relieve symptoms of itching and scaling.

HOMEOPATHY
Acid nit. – eczema of lips, nostrils, anywhere dry skin meets moist.
Ant. crud. – thick scabs with a sticky secretion beneath.
Arsen. alb. – dry skin, itchy, much dandruff. Patient is restless and prefers to be warm.

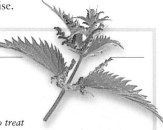

Use nettles to treat allergic eczema.

Borax – eczema of mouth and feet; nails and claws may become loose.
Bovista – eczema of the face and head, severe itching, skin is thickened and bleeds easily. Moist, crusty skin.
Cantharis – burning, itching eczema. Skin very red, sore, and hot.
Graphites – sticky eczema, excessive molting, very smelly skin. Patient likes warmth.
Merc. sol. – wet eczema, sudden onset, gets infected quickly.
Mezereum – scabs with red rings around, under run with pus.
Petroleum – dry, cracked, raw skin.
Psorinum – dirty looking, smelly skin. Patient craves warmth. Good mange remedy.
Rhus tox – itchy, red skin, like nettle rash.
Sulphur – classic homeopathic cooling remedy for hot, itchy skin.
Urtica – for allergic skin rashes.

NUTRITIONAL
Zinc – a good supplement for dry, flaky eczema.
Essential fatty acids (EFAs) – especially evening primrose oil or borage oil with fish oils.
Beetroot juice – a good eczema calming remedy.

STUD TAIL

A condition confined to cats, where it occurs mainly in unneutered males. Stud tail is a greasy secretion on the surface of the upper part of the tail produced from glands below the skin.

The symptoms are a yellow-brown, sticky, greasy secretion, matting the fur on the upper surface of the tail. Some fur loss may occur.

The causes are not known but are presumed to be hormonal, stimulating an overproduction of oil from the skin glands.

To treat it, use the remedies for eczema that are specific for greasy skin and seborrhea. In addition, **tea tree** lotion should be used to clean the affected area twice daily.

Anal gland disorders

The anal glands are scent glands located one on either side of the anus. They produce a secretion, which is normally expressed from the glands when the bowels are emptied. In dogs and cats these glands may become blocked. The secretion builds up inside the glands, causing irritation.

The affected pet may rub its bottom on the floor, turn round and look or chew at the base of the tail, or simply show signs of itchiness anywhere toward the hindquarters. Some dogs will suddenly turn and look at their rear ends as though feeling a shooting pain. Blocked glands (often called impacted glands) are predisposed to infection, and anal gland abscesses are a common consequence of blocked glands, especially in dogs.

The causes are not known, but a lack of fiber in the diet may be a contributory factor, and any treatment should be accompanied by a review of the diet. Anal gland blockage often follows a spell of either constipation or diarrhea, when the glands will not have been emptied naturally.

Treatment involves regular manual emptying of the glands – a job that is probably the single most common procedure carried out by veterinarians! Recurrent problems often result in a suggestion from the vet that the glands should be removed surgically. Before reaching that decision, the following remedies may be successful.

DOS AND DON'TS

Don't try and empty the glands yourself, unless your veterinarian has shown you how to carry out the procedure.

Don't assume itchy bottoms are caused by worms – anal gland blockage is a much more common cause.

Don't ask for a ferret's anal glands to be removed, thinking it will get rid of the natural odor of the ferret. It doesn't!

ABOVE *Ferrets have a strong natural odor – unfortunately anal gland removal will not solve it.*

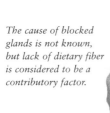

The cause of blocked glands is not known, but lack of dietary fiber is considered to be a contributory factor.

CAUSES

- unknown, but lack of dietary fiber may be a contributory factor

SIGNS AND SYMPTOMS

- pet may chew the base of its tail

REMEDIES

NUTRITIONAL
Ensure there is sufficient fiber and roughage in the diet. Add bran if necessary.

HERBAL
Dandelion – infusions of dandelion petals give gentle help in relieving blocked glands.

HOMEOPATHY
Hepar sulph. – for infected anal glands, painful to touch.
Silicea – a remedy for repeated blockages.
Merc sol. – for thick, greenish discharge from the glands.

Dandelion can be used as an infusion.

Feather and skin conditions in birds

The skin of birds is obviously different from that of mammals; owners of birds need to watch for certain conditions that are specific to feathers, as well as a few actual skin problems.

Symptoms may include ruffled feathers, which are seen at any time when birds are unwell, but do not necessarily imply a feather or skin problem. The bird will often be inactive and other signs of disease may be present. Treat according to the underlying diseases.

FEATHER LOSS

Combined with areas of baldness, this may just be a heavy molt. Alternatively, it could be caused by skin parasites, or may be a nutritional deficiency.

BROKEN FEATHERS

Caused by trauma, perhaps by attacks from other birds, or by human damage. Parasites can weaken feathers so that they break easily when placed under stress.

STUNTED FEATHERS

Stunted growth is caused by parasites or nutritional deficiencies.

SELF PLUCKING

Birds that pluck their own feathers may do so from boredom or other behavioral reasons, or because they are reacting to an irritation from parasites.

PUFFY SWELLINGS OF SKIN

Occasionally a bird will rupture an air sac; air sacs are air pockets which are found in several locations in the bird's body and help keep it light and able to fly. The air from this sac comes to the surface under the skin of neck or chest and causes a puffy swelling.

SOFT SWELLING OF SKIN

Often with loss of the covering feathers. This is caused by abscesses or bruises under the skin, or by fatty cysts called lipomas that can become quite large and affect the bird's ability to fly.

SCALY LEGS OR BEAK

A powdery, scaly appearance to legs (scaly leg) or beak (scaly beak) is usually caused by a mite infestation. The beak can become deformed if the condition progresses.

SWELLING OF SKIN OVER JOINTS OF FEET

Usually caused by a bacterial infection. This can be very painful, and affected birds may have difficulty in grasping and holding onto perches.

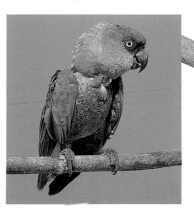

ABOVE *Swelling of the feet is usually a bacterial infection.*

LEFT *Baldness may caused by parasites or inadequate nutrition.*

REMEDIES

Treatment depends on the cause of the condition. Parasites must be eliminated if present. Conventional antiparasite agents will be needed, but these can be backed up by natural remedies, which can also be used to help prevent recurrence of parasites (see pages 162–165). Injuries, bruises, infections, and abscesses will need veterinary attention, but natural medicines will help – see the appropriate section. Attacks from other birds and self-plucking from boredom will need a review of where and how the bird is kept, and the size and position of the cage. Check nutrition is adequate in all cases.

Shell and scales conditions

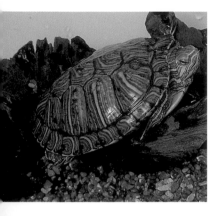

Meat is an essential part of the terrapin diet to stop their shells becoming soft.

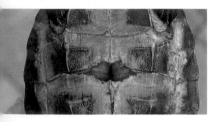

This terrapin has a hole in the center of its shell – an example of trauma commonly suffered by chelonians through human or animal attack.

The scales or shells of reptiles, chelonians (tortoises and terrapins), and fish have their own conditions. The commonest problems are detailed below.

BEAK DEFORMITIES

The hard tissue of the mouth, or beak, of tortoises and terrapins can become deformed as a result of nutritional osteodystrophy, a mineral deficiency caused by incorrect feeding (see Diet, page 13).

REMEDIES: SHELL

Treatment includes necessary veterinary attention, but do also use remedies for wounds and injuries – especially:

HOMEOPATHY
Arnica (by mouth) – for trauma.
Hypericum and **calendula** ointment on the wound.
Cantharis (by mouth) – for burns.

HERBAL
Aloe vera gel applied to the shell wound.

REMEDIES: SCALE

HOMEOPATHY
Hypericum and **calendula** ointment applied to the skin.
Apis mel. (by mouth) to treat and prevent infection.

HERBAL
Aloe vera gel applied to the skin.

SOFT SHELL

All chelonians have soft shells when born. These harden gradually, and a correct balanced diet is necessary for this to take place. Terrapins often suffer from soft shell in adulthood because of insufficient meat in their diet (see Diet, page 13).

SHELL TRAUMA

Shells may be damaged in falls, from getting caught in lawn mowers, from attacks by rodents while hibernating, and from burns while sheltering in piles of rubbish that are then burned by their owners.

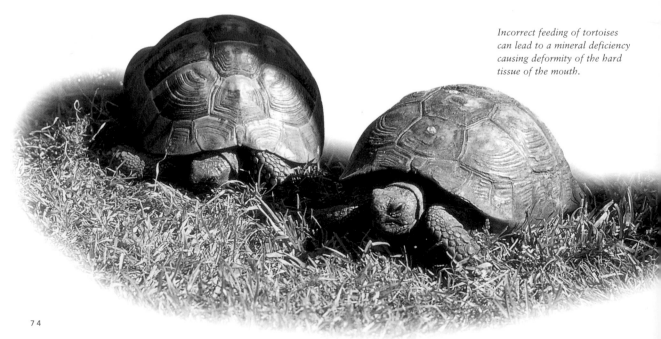

Incorrect feeding of tortoises can lead to a mineral deficiency causing deformity of the hard tissue of the mouth.

Skin and scale disorders

BLISTER DISEASE

A condition of lizards and snakes. Blisters are seen on the skin and may become widespread. Usually caused by parasites; may be secondary bacterial infection. The parasites must be treated; additionally, the remedies below will help heal the blisters. Blister disease occurs more readily in high humidity. Check humidity levels.

SCALE ROT

A condition of snakes where infection penetrates below the scales, causing the scales and underlying skin to die and peel off, leaving raw exposed tissue beneath. This raw tissue is then vulnerable to further infection. It is mainly caused by poor hygiene and environment. Treat as for wounds and injuries; hypericum and calendula ointment are especially good for this. Review and improve environment; if necessary, seek expert advice (see Housing, page 17).

REMEDIES FOR FISH

HOMEOPATHY

Administer homeopathic tablets by dissolving them in the tank water. For further information, see instructions in the chapter on Homeopathy (page 44).

Acid nit. – for ulcer disease.
Bovista – for fin rot.
Petroleum – for ulcer disease.
Mezereum – for fungal diseases.
Psorinum – for parasitic diseases.

DYSECDYSIS

An inability to shed the skin properly. All lizards and snakes shed their skin regularly as they grow. Dysecdysis is caused by too high or low humidity, or an absence of areas to bathe in or rocks to rub against. Prevent this condition by improving the environment. Help a snake to shed its skin by placing wet towels in a box, and put the snake among them – rubbing against the towels will help the shedding process.

FISH DISEASES

Fish are prone to a variety of diseases affecting scales and skin: ulcer disease, fungus, white spot, and fin rot. These are nearly always caused by infections or parasites. In order to treat any of these conditions, it is necessary to isolate the affected fish in a separate tank that has been scrupulously cleaned. Check the condition of the usual tank or aquarium – this is often a factor. Add the appropriate homeopathic remedies, shown on the left, to any necessary conventional treatment.

ABOVE *Fish are prone to a variety of diseases that affect their scales or skin. These are mostly caused by infections or parasites.*

LEFT *Problems with shedding their skin properly is usually caused by incorrect housing.*

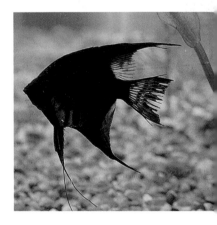

ABOVE *This Angel fish is suffering from fin rot – caused by an infection.*

Otitis externa

This is inflammation of the ear canal and is a typical ear problem in many pets.

The symptoms include head-shaking, scratching the ear, and tenderness. There may be a visible discharge from one or both ears, and an unpleasant smell from the ear.

Otitis externa is not a single condition – there are many possible causes:

• Parasites (ear mites): discharge is often dry and crusty, dark in color, with intense itching. Both ears are usually affected.

• Foreign bodies: commonly grass seeds. The seeds of some grasses have sharp barbs that cause intense pain and irritation when the seed enters the ear canal. One ear is affected, with much head-shaking and ear-scratching.

• Ear growths: polyps or tumors in the ear may block the canal and cause a build-up of wax below the growth. This predisposes to infection developing. Usually in one ear.

• Allergies: some allergic reactions, especially to pollens, cause an itchy, sore ear. In most cases, there is inflammation of other areas – the feet and/or groins, armpits, and

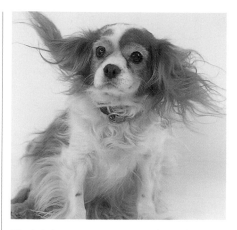

Head-shaking is a common sign of ear infection.

lower abdomen. Usually affects both ears.

• Infections: bacteria and yeast are the commonest infections in ears, causing a discharge, often smelly, with visible pus. May affect one or both ears. Infections often occur as secondary invaders in an ear already inflamed from another cause.

All dog breeds with ears that hang down or with hair within their ears, which reduces air flow, are likely to be affected.

Cloves are a powerful natural antiseptic and analgesic.

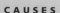

CAUSES

• parasites
• foreign bodies, eg. grass seeds
• ear growths (polyps or tumors)
• allergies
• infection with bacteria or yeast

SIGNS AND SYMPTOMS

• head-shaking
• scratching
• tenderness
• may be discharge
• may be unpleasant smell

REMEDIES

First remove any obvious causes. Polyps may respond to remedies for warts. Tumors in the ear canal may respond to remedies for cancer. Allergic otitis externa should be treated with remedies for eczema, depending on symptoms.

COLOR THERAPY
Indigo is the appropriate color.

AROMATHERAPY
Clove and **thyme** – massage diluted oils into the skin near the ears.

CRYSTAL AND GEM ESSENCES
Diamond – a diamond is an ear's best friend!
Hemimorphite – for thick, waxy, persistent ear secretions and infections.

HERBAL
Rosemary infusion
– (3 parts) with witch hazel (1 part) makes an effective ear cleansing lotion.
Lemon juice – a few drops in 1 teaspoon olive oil is also a good ear cleansing treatment.
Thyme, rosemary, rue infusion, mixed equally with olive oil; an effective treatment for ear mites.

HOMEOPATHY
Calendula – with hypericum lotion for cleansing.
Belladonna – for acute, hot, painful ears.
Hepar. sulph. – for infected, purulent discharge.
Graphites – for sticky, smelly ears.
Merc. corr. – for thick, greenish discharge.
Psorinum – for hot, itchy, smelly ears. Likes warmth.
Sulphur – for hot, itchy ears. Dislikes heat.

Otitis media and interna

These names describe inflammation that occurs beyond the ear drum in the middle or inner parts of the ear.

The symptoms include head-shaking and ear-scratching, although there may be no visible soreness or discharge, as the problem is beyond the ear drum. There may be a head tilt to one side, and in acute cases a loss of balance, or circling in one direction.

The infection is often a progression from otitis externa, so pets may be affected by this condition at the same time. There is usually a spread of infection, either from the ear canal or from the throat. Occasionally these conditions are caused by tumors.

LEFT *A veterinarian will make a thorough investigation of the ear drum and inner ear if otitis is suspected.*

RIGHT *As the infection spreads, it may extend the inflammation and swelling to the ear flap.*

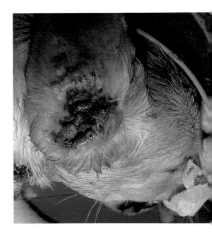

CAUSES

- progression from otitis externa
- tumor

SIGNS AND SYMPTOMS

- head-shaking
- ear-scratching
- head tilt
- loss of balance
- circling in one direction

REMEDIES

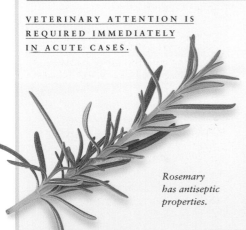

VETERINARY ATTENTION IS REQUIRED IMMEDIATELY IN ACUTE CASES.

Rosemary has antiseptic properties.

AROMATHERAPY
Rosemary and **thyme** (diluted) massaged around the base of the ear.

FLOWER AND GEM REMEDIES
Scleranthus can help loss of balance.

HOMEOPATHY
Hepar. sulph. – where infection is likely to be the cause.
Silicea – in long-standing cases will help clear discharges, and the scarring that forms as a result of the infection.
Belladonna – if there is a fever accompanying the condition.

Aural hematoma

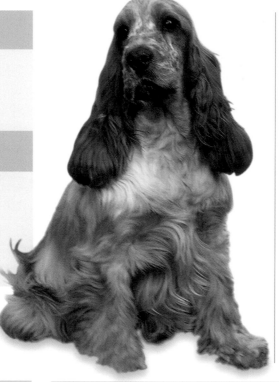

Dog breeds with long pendulous ears are prone to various aural disorders including aural hematoma.

This is a hemorrhage that occurs within the ear flap, causing it to swell.

The symptoms are violent head-shaking, with a rapidly swelling ear flap. The ear flap (pinna) may become enormously swollen and heavy, so that the ear hangs down.

There are various causes.
- Trauma – physical injury.
- Parasites – ear mites are notorious for causing so much irritation that the head-shaking and ear-scratching predisposes to hematoma formation.
- Otitis externa – any type of otitis externa, by making the ear sore and itchy, will predispose to aural hematoma.
- Auto-immune disease – pets with certain types of auto-immune disorders are prone to hemorrhage easily, and so many suffer repeated hematomas.

DOS AND DON'TS

Do use an ice pack if you are present when an ear flap injury occurs (see cold and compression page 59) – cold and pressure may prevent a hematoma occurring.

If your pet develops acute symptoms, do contact your veterinarian as soon as possible.

Don't handle the ear flap more than necessary.

Do try and stop your pet from shaking its head – this will exacerbate the hematoma. Use natural calming agents if necessary.

REMEDIES

Conventional treatment for acute aural hematoma is usually surgical – draining the hemorrhage and then suturing the ear flap to prevent recurrence of the hematoma.
If the condition can be treated while in the early stages, or if the hematoma is developing slowly, natural remedies may be sufficient to avoid the necessity of surgery. Natural medicines can also be used to help heal the ear after surgery, and to reduce the thickening end.

HERBAL
Apply **witch hazel** lotion to the ear flap directly. Use clean, soft, cotton pads. Apply the lotion liberally and discard each pad after use.

HOMEOPATHY
Apis mel. – for rapidly developing swollen, shiny ear flaps.
Cantharis – for the hot, painful, burning feeling.
Arnica – give the acute dosage as soon as the hematoma is noticed, then go on to hamamelis.

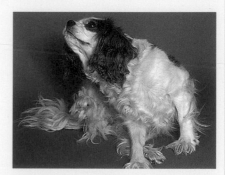

Rapid swelling of the ear will cause discomfort and pronounced head shaking and scratching.

Hamamelis – give at the chronic dosage until the hematoma is reabsorbed and the swelling has gone. This may take some time, but hamamelis can be given for several weeks if necessary.
Silicea – for chronic thickening and scarring of the ear flaps, either following surgery, or following natural shrinkage of the blood clot.

Warts

Warts are skin growths that occur commonly in dogs, occasionally in cats and rarely in other species. They are normally harmless, but can become itchy, which means the pet scratches or bites at them. They may also be prone to repeated bleeding if they are large enough to get knocked or damaged, and can then become infected. In themselves they are not usually a cause for ill health.

Typical warts include growths in the skin, which can be anywhere on the body. Shapes vary from flat (called sessile) to cauliflower-like growths. There may be a stalk attaching the wart to the skin (called a pedunculated wart). Colors vary from pink to black, and they may grow slowly or rapidly. They are caused sometimes as a result of viral infections, but often there is no known cause.

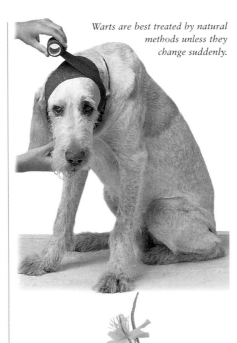

Warts are best treated by natural methods unless they change suddenly.

Greater celandine

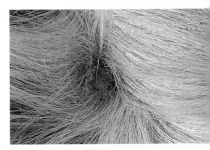

ABOVE *Warts vary in color and shape – this dog has a sessile, pink wart.*

CAUSES

- often unknown, but sometimes due to viral infection

SIGNS AND SYMPTOMS

- growths in the skin
- colors vary from pink to black

REMEDIES

AROMATHERAPY
Lemon – a good general antiwart remedy.
Tagetes – for large, hard warts, and for calluses and thickened skin in general.

FLOWER AND GEM REMEDIES
Coral is a noted wart treatment.

HERBAL
Greater celandine – apply the juice from the plant to the wart daily.
Garlic – apply fresh slices to the wart daily.
Milk thistle – give by infusion.

HOMOEOPATHY
Acid nit. – for warts that are jagged and bleed easily. The warts often seem painful and the affected pet will lick or chew at them. In older animals, there may be accompanying liver or kidney problems.
Ant. crud. – for dry skin with a tendency to multiple wart formation. Warty growths often appear on the skin of the pads of the feet. Eczema may also be noticed.
Calc. carb. – use for flat, round warts. Often in animals that are heavily built and/or overweight.
Causticum – use for warts that are flat, often bleed easily, and are mainly on the face, including eyelids. Particularly suits old, stiff animals.
Thuja – for all warts, especially those that bleed easily. Can be applied as a tincture: one drop on each wart daily.

OTHER TREATMENTS
Taping **banana skin** over a wart can be effective. Cut a square of freshly peeled banana skin, large enough to cover the entire area of the wart, and tape it over the wart, outer skin uppermost. Secure it with with medical adhesive tape (make sure this is not too tight). Replace daily.

DOS AND DON'TS

Do have any rapidly growing wart checked by your veterinarian, or any wart that suddenly changes shape or consistency, or becomes very itchy.

Don't expect treatment to make warts disappear overnight – shrinkage is gradual and sometimes warts will simply stop growing rather than actually shrink.

Conjunctivitis

Conjunctivitis is an inflammation of the pink mucous membrane surrounding the white of the eye.

The symptoms are red, sore-looking eyes, with or without a watery, or thick and purulent discharge, in one or both eyes. The affected pet may rub the eyes, or rub the face in the ground or on other objects.

• Guinea pigs often have conjunctivitis at the same time as respiratory infections, or as a result of hay or straw in the eyes.
• Birds are prone to conjunctivitis. One possible cause is chlamydia – an organism that causes psittacosis, a disease that is transmittable to humans. Always have eye problems in birds checked thoroughly by your veterinarian. There are various causes:
• Foreign bodies – usually in one eye only. The eye can be red and very painful, extremely itchy with a watery discharge.
• Physical injuries.
• Entropion – ingrowing eyelids rub on the eye causing conjunctivitis.
• Distichiasis – ingrowing eyelashes similarly irritate one or both eyes.
• Allergy – some pets sensitive to allergies will develop conjunctivitis as part of the allergic symptoms. Usually affects both eyes.
• Infection – bacteria and viral infections will cause conjunctivitis. In most pets, discharge is usually present. Affects both eyes in most cases, but usually starts in one eye first.

ABOVE *Ingrowing eyelids and eyelashes are a common cause of conjunctivitis.*

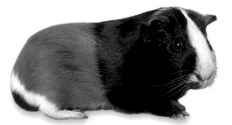

LEFT *Guinea pigs with respiratory infections will often develop conjunctivitis.*

CAUSES

• foreign bodies
• physical injury
• entropion
• distichiasis
• allergy
• bacterial or viral infection

SIGNS AND SYMPTOMS

• violent head-shaking
• red, sore-looking eyes, with or without discharge
• pet may rub its eyes or rub face on the ground

REMEDIES

Treatment for conjunctivitis should be sought quickly; any very sore or very painful eye condition needs rapid attention from your veterinarian. Remove any underlying cause such as a foreign body, and have entropion (ingrowing eyelids) or distichiasis (ingrowing eyelashes) attended to.

COLOR THERAPY
Indigo treats both ear and eye problems.

HERBAL
Greater celandine or **dock infusion** may be used to bathe the eyes up to three times daily. Keep the infusion cool and covered. Make up a fresh supply of the infusion daily.
Vervain compresses – to treat with vervain, soak a cotton pad in a freshly prepared infusion of vervain and apply gentle pressure against the eye for 1–2 minutes three times daily.

HOMEOPATHY
Euphrasia – (Eyebright) tincture. Dilute 3 drops in 2 teaspoons sterile water and bathe the eyes three times daily. Make up fresh solution daily.
Calc. sulph. – for the thick white discharge of rabbit conjunctivitis.
Apis mel. – swollen eyelids or conjunctivitis.
Arsen alb. – watery, acrid discharge.
Kali bich. – thick, green, stringy discharge.
Pulsatilla – creamy, catarrhal discharge.
Aconite – conjunctivitis from cold winds.

CRYSTALS AND GEM ESSENCES
Opal, turquoise, and **topaz** are beneficial.

Topaz gem has a healing effect on eye conditions.

Corneal disease

The cornea is the central, transparent area of the eye. It is a very delicate structure – even a tiny scratch may form an ulcer rapidly. It has no blood supply – if it had blood vessels running through it, these would prevent clear vision. Therefore it heals very slowly – healing agents have to diffuse slowly across the surface, rather than be carried by blood vessels. However, if there is a severe corneal injury, small blood vessels will grow into the cornea to help healing and then shrink and disappear when their job is done.

Two main corneal problems occur in pets – keratitis and corneal ulcers.

KERATITIS

Keratitis is an inflammation of the cornea. The symptoms include a watery eye and rapid blinking of the eyes. As the condition increases, the cornea becomes opaque and reduces vision.

It is caused by infections (bacterial, viral, and fungal), trauma (physical injuries), foreign bodies (grass seeds and splinters in the eye), and immune system disease.

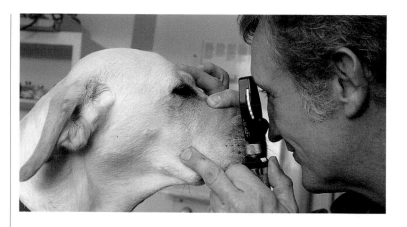

CORNEAL ULCER

A corneal ulcer is an ulceration of the corneal tissue. The symptoms are as keratitis, but more acute. Photophobia (when the pet cannot tolerate bright light) is also common.

The causes are also as keratitis: trauma, entropion, dry eye. Ulcers are often at the center of the cornea and usually affect one eye only, but occasionally will be seen in both eyes. They are serious – they can penetrate the cornea and cause eye damage and blindness. Rapid veterinary attention is essential.

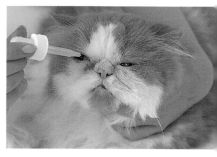

ABOVE TOP *Always seek veterinary advice if your pet develops corneal ulcers.*

ABOVE *Remedies can be administered directly onto the cornea using a dropper.*

REMEDIES

When treating keratitis and corneal ulcers, first ensure that any underlying problem is treated – foreign bodies removed, entropion or distichiasis corrected. Avoid exposing pets with corneal ulcers to bright light.

HERBAL
Greater celandine infusion – bathe the eye four to five times daily. Keep the infusion cool and covered; make up a fresh supply daily.

HOMEOPATHY
Euphrasia tincture – 3 drops in 2 teaspoons sterile water. Bathe the eye four to five times daily. Keep cool and covered; make up fresh daily.
Argent nit. – for keratitis and ulcers, with pain and photophobia.
Silicea – for the scarring and opacity during or after corneal disease.
Calc. fluor. – for keratitis.
Ledum – for ulcers caused by penetrating injuries.
Natrum mur. – swollen eyelids, watery discharge, corneal ulcers.

NUTRITIONAL
Vitamin A will help heal keratitis and ulcers (essential for terrapins).

CAUSES

- trauma
- entropion
- dry eye
- infection

SIGNS AND SYMPTOMS

- watery eye
- rapid blinking
- inflammation

Cataracts

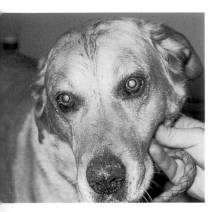

As cataracts develop, the lens of the eye becomes opaque with a bluish discoloration.

These are opacities of the lens, the part of the eye that focuses the light passing through it on to the retina. The lens must be transparent to let light travel through it. Therefore any opacity that develops will reduce vision and eventually cause partial or complete blindness.

The symptoms are visible bluish or white discoloration of the lens in the eye, and visual impairment (bumping into things, hesitant when on walks).

• Cataracts can be congenital, or may develop as an aging process.

• They often form in diabetic pets.

• Eye injuries and infection can precipitate cataracts.

• They are commonest in dogs, sometimes seen in cats, and only occasionally seen in smaller pets. Tortoises sometimes develop cataracts, and may have to be hand-fed, although, with appropriate help and training, they will usually learn to take food even if they cannot see it.

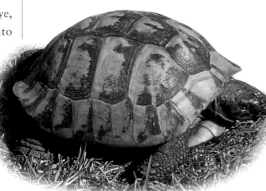

Tortoises with cataracts have reduced vision. This can prevent them from seeing their food.

CAUSES

• may be congenital or due to aging
• diabetes
• injury of infection

SIGNS AND SYMPTOMS

• bluish/white discoloration of the lens of the eye
• visual impairment

DOS AND DON'TS

Don't expect rapid change – the likeliest result with treatment is simply no further deterioration, rather than actual improvement.

REMEDIES

Apart from surgical removal, which has a variable success rate, there is no conventional treatment for cataracts. However, natural medicines can help to slow down or even stop cataract development.

COLOR THERAPY
Yellow slows down cataract formation.

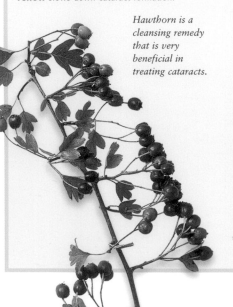

Hawthorn is a cleansing remedy that is very beneficial in treating cataracts.

FLOWER AND GEM REMEDIES
Hawthorn – good for early cataracts.
Sugar beet – helps prevent formation of cataracts in diabetic pets.

CRYSTALS AND GEM ESSENCES
Amethyst should always be used for older pets with cataracts.

HOMEOPATHY
Calc. carb. – for cataracts in large, overweight pets. Cataracts develop slowly, particularly in older animals becoming stiff and arthritic.
Calc. fluor. – for very visible, white cataracts. Often accompanied by poor dental condition.
Conium – for cataracts in old, weakened animals, especially with poor use of the hindquarters.
Phosphorus – for cataracts in thinner, older pets.
Natrum mur. – for recently developed cataracts.

NUTRITIONAL
Vitamin E will help slow down cataract development.

Glaucoma

Glaucoma is an increase in pressure inside the eyeball. The fluid that fills the eyeball is constantly drained and secreted. Normally the rate of secretion of the fluid equals the rate of discharge, so that the pressure of fluid remains constant. If anything disturbs this balance, pressure can build up inside the eye, with a risk of damage to the internal structures of the eye. This can become irreversible, and blindness can eventually result.

The symptoms are an extremely painful eye which may be visibly swollen. The eye will look red and sore, and there may be a watery discharge.

REMEDIES

In addition to any conventional veterinary treatment, try the following.

HOMEOPATHY
Belladonna – for pain and acute inflammation.
Phosphorus – for the inflammation and destruction of internal tissues.
Euphrasia – tincture (diluted by adding 3 drops to 2 teaspoons of sterile water, used 3 times daily) to soothe the eye.

FLOWER AND GEM REMEDIES
Rescue remedy to ease the shock and distress of glaucoma.

CAUSES

- congenital abnormality
- infection
- inflammation
- tumor

SIGNS AND SYMPTOMS

- red, sore eye
- watery discharge
- pet in clear pain

Glaucoma may be caused as a result of a congenital abnormality in the drainage mechanism of the eyeball, or may be the result of infection, inflammation, or tumor in the eye. Symptoms usually occur in one eye first, but the other eye is often affected soon afterward.

Glaucoma is a very serious condition and rapid veterinary attention is required if it occurs or is suspected.

A healthy, happy pet needs good eyesight – ensure it receives a nutritious diet, and consider giving vitamin or mineral supplements.

EPIPHORA

Epiphora is an overflow of tears and occurs mainly with dogs and cats. The symptoms are wet tear stains at the inner corner of the eyes. In light-colored pets, this is obvious as a black or rusty stain.

It is caused by over-production of tears (in conditions such as conjunctivitis or corneal ulcer) and deficient drainage of tears, usually because of blocked drainage ducts. Treat any underlying cause, such as conjunctivitis. Keep animal away from dusty environments, which can aggravate symptoms.

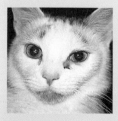

The blocked tear ducts of epiphora cause an over-production of tears, making wet tear stains that discolor.

HOMEOPATHY
Clean and bathe eyes regularly with Euphrasia tincture – 3 drops in 2 teaspoons sterile water; bathe eyes daily. Make up fresh solution daily.
Allium cepa. – for runny, watery eyes, and mucoid discharge.
Natrum mur. – for watery, acrid tears, leaving raw skin in the tracks of the tears.

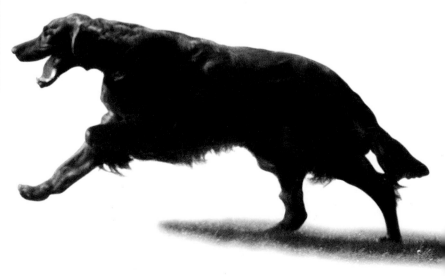

Entropion, distichiasis, and ectropion

CAUSES

- turning-in of eyelid
- presence of extra ingrowing eyelashes
- turning-out of eyelid

SIGNS AND SYMPTOMS

- sore, red eye
- may be discharge

Entropion is a turning-in of one or more eyelids. Distichiasis is the presence of extra ingrowing eyelashes. Ectropion is a turning-out of one or more eyelids.

These three conditions all cause conjunctivitis, either because of the irritation to the eye caused by the lids or lashes rubbing on the eye, or because the turning-out of ectropion lets dust and debris collect in the eye and affects natural tear drainage – also causing irritation and soreness. The affected eye becomes sore and red, and may discharge.

All these problems are congenital, and almost solely found in dogs. Certain breeds are more likely to be affected – for instance, Shar Peis are particularly prone to suffer entropion, spaniels to distichiasis, and bloodhounds to ectropion. If the problem is not corrected, more severe eye problems such as corneal ulceration may develop as a result. The natural remedies below may give some relief. Surgical correction may be necessary and, unfortunately, the conditions do tend to recur in some individuals.

REMEDIES

In addition to any surgical or other treatment, try the following.

HOMEOPATHY
Borax – will help encourage eyelids to uncurl in cases of entropion.
Euphrasia tincture (3 drops in 2 teaspoons sterile water; bathe eyes 3 times daily). Keep cool and covered, and make up solution fresh daily. This will soothe sore eyes.

Bathing the eye with an infusion of rosemary will bring relief.

HERBAL
Rosemary – infusion will help relieve the soreness caused by these conditions.

Shar Peis, spaniels, and bloodhounds – right to left – are more vulnerable to eye afflictions owing to their heavy-lidded appearance.

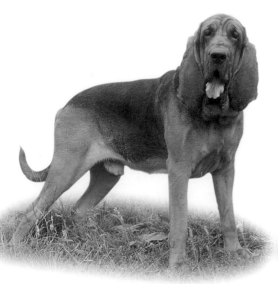

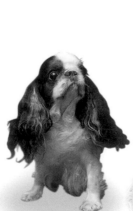

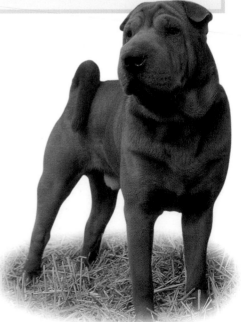

Uveitis

This is an inflammation of the tissues inside the eye, in particular the iris, the colored part of the eye.

The symptoms are pain; photophobia; watery eyes; visibly thickened iris, or color change of the iris in cats; constricted pupil; and pus in the eye.

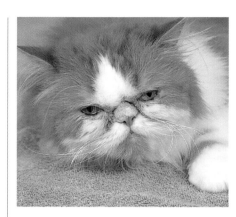

It is often caused by immune system damage, but can also be caused by eye injuries. Infections can bring about uveitis as a secondary effect, as can some kinds of cancer. The most likely of such causes are: canine hepatitis and lymphosarcoma in dogs; feline leukemia virus and feline coronavirus (FIP); toxoplasmosis in cats.

REMEDIES

In addition to necessary conventional veterinary treatment, try:

HOMOEOPATHY
Phosphorus – for bleeding and destruction of tissues in the eyeball.
Rhus tox. – for general inflammation and irritation in the eye.
Symphytum – where uveitis is a result of injury to the eyes.

CAUSES

• immune system damage
• injury
• infection
• cancer

SIGNS AND SYMPTOMS

• pain
• photophobia
• watery eyes
• thickened iris
• constricted pupil
• pus in the eye

Uveitis in cats will cause pain with watery eyes, a visibly thickened iris or a color change in the iris, a constricted pupil, and pus in the eye.

Dry eye

This is a deficiency in the production of tears. The symptoms include: visibly dry and dull eye; cloudy cornea; sticky, thick, mucoid discharge that is prone to infection; dry nose; soreness and irritation of eyes.

Once again, causes of dry eye are often associated with immune system disease. Many cases are caused by an auto-immune disorder, where the normal tear-producing glands are damaged.

Accidents and injuries to the eye can cause dry eye; in cats, feline herpes virus can cause symptoms of dry eye. Treatment with the conventional drug Salazopyrin, an anti-colitis medicine, can cause the condition; tear production should be regularly tested while using this drug.

REMEDIES

Long-term treatment with eye medication or even surgical treatment may be necessary. Natural remedies relieve symptoms effectively.

COLOR THERAPY
Indigo is beneficial.

HOMEOPATHY
Zinc met. – for sore, dry, sticky eyes.
Silicea – for the scarring caused by dry eye.
Conium – for dry eye in old, weak dogs.
Kali bich. – for dry eye with green, discharge.
Euphrasia – for sticky mucus on cornea. Give by mouth, or as tincture.
Cineraria – used as a lotion to bathe the eyes.
Hepar sulph. – when infection is developing in the eyes.

CAUSES

• immune system disease
• accident or injury
• feline herpes virus
• Salazopyrin treatment

SIGNS AND SYMPTOMS

• visibly dry and dull
• cloudy cornea
• sticky mucoid discharge
• dry nose
• soreness and irritation of eyes

Dental Disease and salivary cyst

CAUSES

- injury
- infection
- poor diet
- poor oral hygiene

SIGNS AND SYMPTOMS

- pain and discomfort when eating
- loose or damaged teeth
- tartar on the teeth
- drooling thick, smelly saliva

Unfortunately, many pets will show no outward sign of dental problems for some time; by the time symptoms are noticeable, the disease may be advanced. It is vital to check pets' teeth regularly – at least once a week – for signs of dental disease.

The symptoms include: pain and discomfort when eating; loose or visibly damaged teeth; bad breath; visible tartar on the teeth; drooling, thick, smelly saliva.

The principal causes are:
- Injuries – causing cracked or broken teeth.
- Infection – bacteria cause secondary infection with tartar and gum inflammation.

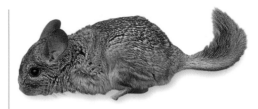

The teeth in small mammals continue growing and are kept in check by constant gnawing.

- Poor diet – the main cause of dental disease in domestic animals.
- Poor oral hygiene – not brushing the teeth!
- In smaller pets, teeth grow continuously and wear naturally by rubbing against each other. If the teeth do not meet properly, they do not wear, and overgrow. The affected animal cannot eat properly, will drool saliva, and the overgrown teeth can be seen. These teeth will need to be trimmed regularly.

SALIVARY CYST

This is cystic swelling in the salivary gland. Its symptom is a soft facial swelling, gradually increasing in size. The causes of this condition are unknown.

REMEDIES: DENTAL DISEASE

To treat dental disease, the damaged teeth may need to be removed. Overgrown teeth in small pets will need to be trimmed. Be sure to choose an appropriate diet – pets on a natural diet have few, if any, dental problems. For dogs and cats, a raw meat diet with raw bones to gnaw and chew, is ideal. Otherwise, choose a diet with hard, crunchy ingredients. For all animals, brush teeth regularly.

AROMATHERAPY
German camomile is good for the nerve pains of toothache and teething.

CRYSTAL AND GEM ESSENCES
Amber and **jet** both relieve dental pain and discomfort.

HOMEOPATHY
Fragaria – helps reduce build-up of plaque on teeth.
Calc. fluor. – strengthens teeth and jaws.
Hepar sulph. – for infections in tooth roots.
Merc. sol. – for the bad breath and salivation.
Hypericum – for painful mouths.
Kreosotum – for rapidly decaying teeth and mouth infections.

NUTRITIONAL
Rubbing **strawberry juice** on the teeth helps keep them clean and free of tartar.

Make sure your pet has its teeth cleaned regularly.

REMEDIES: SALIVARY CYST

To treat salivary cysts, surgical drainage may be required, but healing is very prolonged. Hamsters may develop a swollen face – this is not due to a salivary cyst but to food stuck in the cheek pouch. Empty and flush gently with lukewarm water.

HOMEOPATHY
Apis mel. – if the swelling is very soft and pits on pressure (leaves a small depression which takes a few seconds to refill).
Phytolacca – for firmer swellings.
Silicea – for later stages, when the swelling has hardened, or scarring is present.

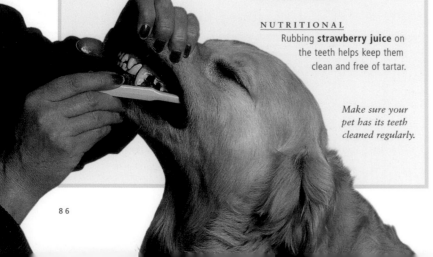

Gingivitis and stomatitis

Gingivitis is an inflammation of the gums; stomatitis is an inflammation of the lining of the mouth. They often occur together. It is important to remove any diseased or damaged teeth and treat an underlying condition, such as kidney disease, which is a factor in the development of gingivitis or stomatitis.

There are many symptoms, some of which include mouth ulcers, discomfort when eating, and pain on opening and closing the mouth.

Bacterial infection is the commonest cause, but infection may be secondary to other causes such as lead poisoning or diabetes, splinters in the mouth, and immune system disorders.

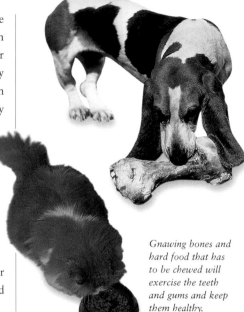

Gnawing bones and hard food that has to be chewed will exercise the teeth and gums and keep them healthy.

CAUSES

- bacterial infection
- lead poisoning
- diabetes

SIGNS AND SYMPTOMS

- mouth ulcers
- dicomfort when eating
- pain on opening the mouth

REMEDIES

Treat both with the following:

AROMATHERAPY
Bergamot – an excellent remedy to soothe inflamed gums and mouth.
Clove bud – a healing oil for bruised and sore gums.
Cypress – helps treat infected gums, also relieves the mental distress of a sore mouth.

HOMEOPATHY
Agnus castus – healing agent for mouth ulcers.
Argent nit. – for sore ulcerated mouths. Affected pet may also have digestive upsets, with vomiting.

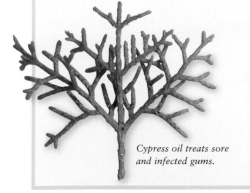

Cypress oil treats sore and infected gums.

Borax – blister-like ulcers in the mouth. Sore eyes or feet may also be present.
Camomile – for the sore gums caused by teething in young puppies and kittens. Often a greenish diarrhea at the same time.
Hepar sulph. – for infected gums with purulent discharge.
Kali chlor. – mouth ulcers, bad breath, and thick, acrid saliva – usually caused by kidney disease.
Kreosotum – mouth infection with decaying teeth.
Merc. corr. – mouth ulcers with thick saliva, increased thirst.
Phosphorus – gums which bleed easily, bright red color.
Plumbum met. – swollen gums with a blue discoloration.

NUTRITIONAL
Coenzyme Q10 will always help to heal gingivitis.
Vitamin C stimulates healing. Vitamin C on one day, alternating with garlic the next, is a good combination for long-standing gingivitis.
Vitamin A also stimulates healing of chronic gingivitis.

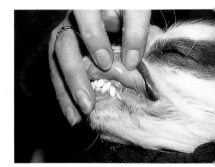

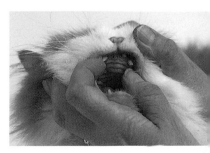

ABOVE TOP *Gingivitis is commonly caused by bacterial infection.*

ABOVE *Broken teeth can lead to infection and disease in the mouth and gums.*

Pharyngitis

CAUSES

- foreign bodies
- infection
- spread of gingivitis and stomatitis
- swallowing of poison
- spread of upper respiratory tract disease

SIGNS AND SYMPTOMS

- poor appetite
- excessive salvation
- difficulty in breathing
- retching
- vomiting
- coughing

Pharyngitis is, in essence, a sore throat. The pharynx is part of both the digestive system (mouth meeting throat) and respiratory system (throat meeting larynx and windpipe). Problems in either of these can cause disease of the pharynx.

Infections of the pharynx are seen in all species, often as a spread from mouth or respiratory infection – such as mouth rot in tortoises or respiratory infection in snakes. Birds may be affected by food lodged in the crop. This is treated as for pharyngitis.

Symptoms include poor appetite, excessive salvation, difficulty in breathing easily, retching or vomiting, and coughing.

Causes include:

- Foreign bodies stuck in the throat.
- Infections – bacterial, fungal, or viral.
- Spread of gingivitis and stomatitis (see page 87).
- Spread of upper respiratory tract disease.
- Swallowing of irritant poisons.
- Dogs chasing sticks may catch them end on so that they become lodged in the throat, causing acute pharyngitis.
- Similarly, dogs accompanying anglers can get fish hooks stuck in throats.
- Grass seed and stems can become lodged in tonsils or pharynx, causing pharyngitis.

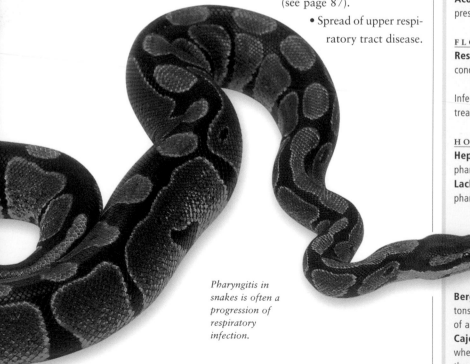

Pharyngitis in snakes is often a progression of respiratory infection.

Treat pharyngitis by removing any predisposing causes, such as foreign bodies. It is difficult to examine the back of the throat of most animals easily, and the affected pet may need to be sedated or anesthetized to see clearly if a foreign body is present – this is a veterinary procedure. After removal of foreign body, give:

HOMEOPATHY
Arnica – for bruising and swelling.
Aconite – for the shock associated with the presence and removal of the foreign body.

FLOWERS AND GEM REMEDIES
Rescue remedy – for the shock and stress of the condition and/or treatment.

Infection may need appropriate conventional treatment. In addition, try:

HOMEOPATHY
Hepar sulph. – for general infection of the pharynx.
Lachesis – for the painful, purplish, swollen pharynx of acute pharyngitis.

Natural remedies for general pharyngitis, and sore throats caused by irritant chemicals:

AROMATHERAPY
Bergamot – for pharyngitis with bad breath and tonsillitis, often with mouth infection. Marked loss of appetite.
Cajeput – for pharyngitis with catarrh, usually where there has been a spread of infection from the respiratory system – sinusitis, flu, and so on.

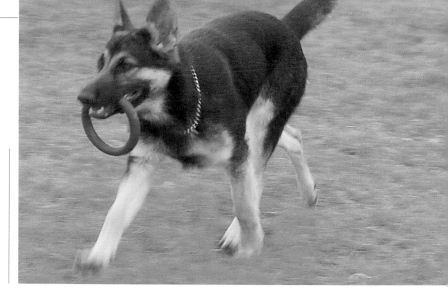

Many pets are unwilling or unable to eat when suffering from acute pharyngitis. Ensure plenty of fluids are available and encourage them to eat soft food in small amounts. Ensure food is strong-smelling (garlic is a good choice and is also an antiseptic), as pharyngitis may be accompanied by sinusitis and a loss of smell.

REMEDIES

Frankincense – for pharyngitis occurring as a spread from bronchitis, laryngitis, or asthma. Frankincense slows down breathing rate, which can help relieve the tension of a sore throat.
Hyssop – for sore throats accompanied by persistent coughing or asthma. DO NOT USE ON EPILEPTIC ANIMALS.
Blue gum eucalyptus – for throat infections, especially as a result of immune system breakdown.
Spanish sage – for pharyngitis with coughing and laryngitis.

CRYSTAL AND GEM ESSENCES
Blue lace agate – for repeated throat infections, especially with an underlying immune problem.
Cat's eye – for pharyngitis of all kinds, and especially for cancer of the throat.
Topaz – for sore throats with loss of voice or change of voice tone (usually a hollow, hoarse sound to the voice).

HOMEOPATHY
Acid nit. – where the throat is bright red and sore, and there appear to be sudden short-lived pains in the throat. In humans, the feeling is as if splinters were being stuck in the throat.
Belladonna – for acute, painful swollen throats. Often a fever, and the affected pet becomes hot, angry, and ready to bite or strike.
Borax – mouth ulcers and throat ulcers, together with a tendency to be scared of noise, and of downward movement.
Ferrum phos. – for sudden-onset red, sore throats.

Blue lace reduces pain and prevents repeated sore throat.

ABOVE *Rubber rings or other toys are better for "fetching" games – sticks can get caught in the throat, causing soreness.*

RIGHT *Cage birds may show symptons similar to pharyngitis when they have food lodged in their crop.*

Kali chlor. – excessive salivation with ulceration. May be kidney disease at the same time.
Baryta carb. – for young dogs with sore throat and swollen glands.
Phytolacca – painful sore throat with enlarged, hardened lymph glands.
Ignatia – for painful, constricted throat, in nervous, anxious patients.

FLOWERS AND GEM REMEDIES
Star of Bethlehem Bach Flower will help relax a tense, sore throat.

NUTRITIONAL
Pineapple juice soothes sore throats and is a good healing agent. DON'T GIVE TO DIABETIC ANIMALS.
Vitamin C is most effective in accelerating healing, fighting infection, and boosting the immune system when treating pharyngitis.
Honey and **garlic**, by mouth, are jointly effective in soothing sore throats and at the same time acting as an antiseptic and freeing the mouth and throat from infection. Alternatively mix 1 teaspoon lemon juice with a little honey and feed this mixture twice daily.

(Inflamed throats caused by poisons should always be referred to a professional.)

DOS AND DON'TS

Do warm the food gently. This brings out natural appetizing odors and makes the food easier to eat.

Do take care when dosing animals with pharyngitis or mouth disease as the mouth may be uncomfortable to open, and the throat tender with pain on swallowing.

Do check the mouth and throat for any signs of foreign bodies. Get veterinary attention if in doubt.

Coughing

CAUSES

- irritants such as cigarette smoke
- fur balls
- infection
- allergies
- lung congestion
- lung hemorrhage
- foreign bodies
- parasites
- cancer
- tracheal collapse
- laryngeal paralysis

SIGNS AND SYMPTOMS

- cough may be productive (mucus is coughed up) or non-productive

The lining of the throat, windpipe, and lungs are delicate, and any irritation or inflammation of these tissues is likely to cause coughing.

Some species and breeds are prone to particular conditions that cause coughing: birds are prone to coughs caused by airborne irritants such as cigarette smoke; cats that are coughing and retching may be trying to bring up fur balls (hair balls).

The cough may be productive – mucus (phlegm) is coughed up; or non-productive – a reflex reaction to an irritant. Coughing has many and various causes:

• Irritants – cigarette smoke is the most common cause.

• Infections – viral, bacterial, or fungal.

• Allergies – these can trigger coughing, with or without other symptoms.

• Lung congestion – excess fluid in the tissues of the lungs will cause a cough. This is often due to heart disease and causes the so-called "heart cough" in many older animals.

• Lung hemorrhage – bleeding into the lungs cause coughing, and obviously blood is coughed up.

• Foreign bodies – all kinds of foreign bodies can be accidentally breathed in. Coughing is a natural protective mechanism in these cases and need not indicate serious illness. However, foreign material, such as liquids that have been inhaled into the lungs

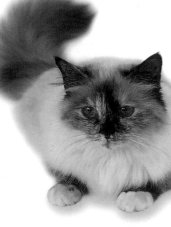

A cat that is repeatedly coughing or retching may have fur balls.

REMEDIES

To treat a cough, remove or stop any obvious causes. Treat parasites and heart disease if either is a cause.

AROMATHERAPY
Angelica root – coughs and colds in general (usually best given via a diffuser).
Benzoin – allergic causes of coughs, coughing with laryngitis and voice loss.
Cajeput – coughing from sore throat or allergic causes.
Elemi – non-productive coughs.
Eucalyptus – asthmatic and catarrhal coughs.
Hyssop – severe coughing such as kennel cough, often with tonsillitis.
Marjoram – asthmatic coughs.
Melissa – chronic, persistent coughing.
Myrrh – catarrhal, croaky coughs, sometimes with loss of voice.
Rosemary – coughs caused by infections, allergies, or by parasites.
Sage (clary) – coughs caused by infections, with sore throats.
Sandalwood – dry, persistent coughs, often with laryngitis.
Tea tree – coughing with catarrh, sinusitis; much mucus production.

FLOWER AND GEM REMEDIES
Topaz – for severe, painful coughs.
Pearl – for catarrhal, productive coughs.
Sage – for heart coughs.

HERBAL
Marshmallow – for irritating, dry non-productive coughs.
Eucalyptus – for chesty coughs and catarrh.
Garlic – for coughs caused by infections or parasites. Helps clear mucus and catarrh.
Liquorice – for irritable, dry coughs.

Licorice is soothing and anti-inflammatory.

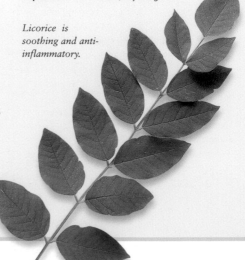

can set up a major inflammation known as inhalation pneumonia, with severe coughing.

• Parasites – various ones can invade the respiratory tract and cause persistent coughing.

• Cancer – tumors growing in or near the respiratory tract can trigger coughing because of the pressure they exert on airways.

• Tracheal collapse – a weakened trachea may partially collapse, and result in frequent bouts of coughing.

• Laryngeal paralysis – weakening of the muscles of the larynx causes coughing in older dogs.

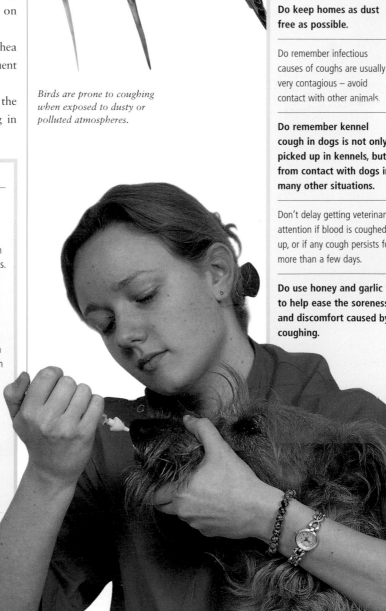

Birds are prone to coughing when exposed to dusty or polluted atmospheres.

HOMEOPATHY

Ant tart. – coughing with an audible wheezy chest, though no mucus is actually coughed up.

Arsen alb. – coughing and wheezing; the cough is often worse at night, and the patient is restless.

Bryonia – dry cough. Coughing tends to be aggravated by movement. Affected pets will not tend to cough while asleep or at rest, but will cough as soon as they get up and start moving.

Drosera – spasmodic, dry cough, with retching or sometimes vomiting. The cough is worse when the patient gets excited, or very active. The cough usually sounds as if caused by something stuck in the throat, and the throat looks red and sore. Ideal for kennel cough in dogs.

Lycopodium – irritating cough, often worse in the afternoon and early evening.

Lycopus – coughs with wheezy breathing; heart disease is usually present.

Spongia tosta – ideal for the "heart cough" – congested lungs, and coughing is worse with exercise.

Vaccination is an effective method of protecting against kennel cough – but remember their are also natural ways of stimulating the immune system.

Nasal discharge and sinusitis

CAUSES

- infection
- spread of abscessation from roots of teeth
- foreign bodies
- tumor or polyp

SIGNS AND SYMPTOMS

- sneezing
- discharge
- difficulty in breathing
- head-shaking

DOS AND DON'TS

Do check environment – temperature, humidity, ventilation – in all cases of sinusitis.

Don't smoke or use aerosol sprays near pets with sinus problems.

Do use humidifiers and ionizers where appropriate.

Aromatherapy by steam inhalation is an excellent method of clearing catarrh and mucus to relieve congestion.

Blocked and congested sinuses, catarrh, and discharges from the nostrils occur in almost all types of pets.

The symptoms are sneezing, discharge from one or both nostrils, difficulty in breathing easily, head-shaking.

The causes may be: infections – bacterial, fungal, or viral; spread of abscessation from roots of teeth; foreign bodies, such as grass seeds or grass stems, inhaled into the nasal passages; tumors or polyps in nasal passages.

REMEDIES

Apart from any necessary veterinary treatment, the following remedies will help clear catarrh and mucus.

Eucalyptus is an effective decongestant.

AROMATHERAPY
Sweet Orange – cold and flu symptoms, especially after being chilled, or being out in wet weather.
Pine needle – catarrh, sinusitis, sore throats. A good strengthening remedy for the weakness that often accompanies chronic sinusitis.
Sandalwood – catarrh, often with a dry, persistent cough.
Hyssop – catarrh, often with tonsillitis and sore throat.
Eucalyptus – ideal for all catarrh and sinusitis sufferers.
Myrrh – colds, catarrh, often with loss of voice.

CRYSTAL AND GEM ESSENCES
Lapis lazuli – for the discomfort of congestion.

HERBAL
Garlic – for all respiratory symptoms.
Licorice – for catarrh with dry coughs.

HOMEOPATHY
Pulsatilla – bland, creamy, catarrhal discharge.
Natrum mur. – watery discharge, much sneezing.
Acid nit. – sore nose with ulcerations, sneezing.
Kali bich. – yellow, thick, stringy discharge.
Allium cepa – running nose and eyes. Hay fever.
Silicea – persistent, chronic sinusitis.

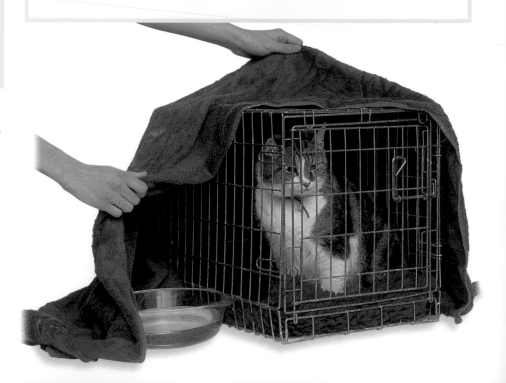

Asthma

Asthma affects the respiratory tract and is an allergic reaction to various allergens, often house dust or smoke.

Its symptoms are: difficulty in breathing; wheezing sounds; congested lungs; and poor oxygenation of blood, which in some cases may lead to bluish discoloration of gums and skin.

Many different allergens can cause asthma – pollens, house dust mites, grasses. Some pets may be reacting to more than one allergen. Certain crops grown by farmers are particularly likely to trigger asthma and produce symptoms similar to those found in hay fever.

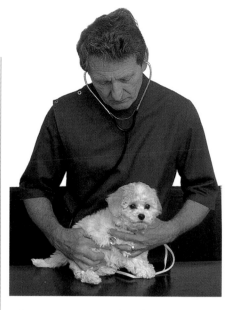
Ask your veterinarian to check lung congestion.

CAUSES

- allergens – for example pollens, house dust mites, grasses

SIGNS AND SYMPTOMS

- difficulty in breathing
- wheezing sounds
- congested lungs
- bluish color of gums and skin

REMEDIES

The following remedies will relieve symptoms of asthma.

AROMATHERAPY
Clary sage – for asthma with frequent coughing.
Cypress – for asthma with spasmodic, intermittent coughing.
Benzoin – for asthma with laryngitis, pronounced wheezing.
Rose maroc – hay fever-like symptoms.
Clove bud – asthma and bronchitis.
Hyssop – asthma with catarrh and sore throat.
Lavender – sore throats, bad breath, and a tendency to asthmatic symptoms.
Sweet marjoram – asthma and all other respiratory symptoms.
Cajeput – sinusitis and asthma.
Lime – for persistent mild asthmatic conditions.
Frankincense – coughs, colds, asthma; and flu.

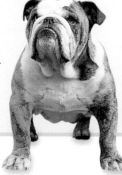
Some breeds of dog, such as the Bulldog, are prone to wheezing and breathing problems.

FLOWER AND GEM REMEDIES
Pearl – either in the liquid gem remedy, or as the gem itself, is an effective asthma remedy.

HERBAL
Garlic – will help relieve asthma (and all respiratory) symptoms.
Vervain – a good asthma remedy, and a strengthening remedy to help counter the debility that asthma often causes.

HOMEOPATHY
Apis mel: – severe lung congestion, often a strong desire for fresh air, noticeable wheezing and difficulty in breathing. There may be visible edema (tissues swollen with fluid) of face or legs.
Arsen alb. – wheezing, labored breathing, with much restlessness, and thirst for small amounts of water, drunk little and often.
Sulfur – asthma with eczema at the same time. Affected patient dislikes heat and looks for cool places to lie.
Spongia tosta – asthma with much coughing and wheezing.
Aspidosperma – used as the tincture. One drop of tincture on the tongue every few minutes will help improve breathing in serious cases of asthma.

DOS AND DON'TS

Do improve ventilation, avoid a dry atmosphere, and avoid any pollutants in the environment, such as smoke, aerosol sprays, or carpet fresheners.

Don't expose an affected pet to wet or cold conditions.

Do give vitamin B supplements, which help symptoms.

Don't assume coughing and wheezing pets necessarily have asthma – heart conditions or other causes may be involved. Any persistent respiratory symptoms must always have veterinary attention.

Epistaxis

Epistaxis is the medical term for nose bleeds. There may be a frequent, or constant flow of blood, or the nose bleeds may be few and far between.

Nose bleeds are caused by:

• Foreign bodies – grass seeds, blades of grass, and so on. In these cases, the bleeding is usually from one nostril only.

• Trauma – accidents and injuries.

• Sneezing – violent sneezing in pets with flu or sinusitis can trigger a nose bleed.

• Infections – particularly aspergillosis, a fungal infection that erodes the lining of the nasal passages and sinuses and leads to frequent nose bleeds.

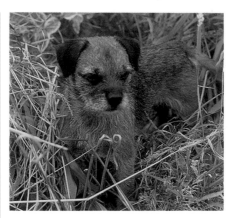

LEFT *Grass and plant seeds and even blades of grass can cause nose bleeds, although it is usually restricted to one nostril.*

BELOW *Bloodstone is a useful remedy for all hemorrhages. It is easily administered as a gem essence.*

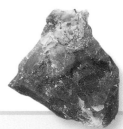

• Tumors – some tumors will also erode the membrane lining nasal passages, and result in nose bleeds.

CAUSES

• foreign bodies
• trauma
• sneezing
• infection
• tumor

SIGNS AND SYMPTOMS

• nose bleeds may be presenyas a frequent or constant flow of blood

Lemon and lime essential oils are very helpful.

REMEDIES

For acute, major nose bleeds, emergency treatment, including cauterizing, may be necessary. Natural medicines that will help include:

AROMATHERAPY

Lemon and lime – both excellent essential oils, which help to minimize nose bleeds, especially in patients that also have a poor circulation, have excess fluid in body tissues, tend to be overweight, and are prone to arthritis.

FLOWER AND GEM REMEDIES

Sapphire – for nose bleeds that are persistent though not necessarily of great volume: a slow but constant trickle.

CRYSTAL AND GEM ESSENCES

Bloodstone – as its name suggests, a remedy for all hemorrhages, including nose bleeds.
Ruby – for nose bleeds of bright red blood.

HOMEOPATHY

Phosphorus – for sudden nose bleeds, or for persistent nose bleeds, where the blood does not clot quickly. Especially useful for nose bleeds that occur as a result of destruction of the bony structure of the nasal passages. This is often caused by a tumor, or by aspergillosis. The patient that needs phosphorus is usually thin and in poor condition, with a fear of sudden bangs and noises.

Hamamelis – for nose bleeds of dark, thick blood that does not clot easily. Eyes may look bloodshot.

Arnica – for nose bleeds caused by accidents and injuries.

Acid nit. – soreness and ulceration of nostrils leading to cracked and fissured nasal area. An acrid, corrosive discharge begins to form, which is often bloodstained. Sneezing is often a feature, and the sneezing may trigger nose bleeds.

Aconite – bright red nosebleeds, often caused by violent sneezing, especially after pet has been exposed to cold, dry, windy weather.

Ferrum phos. – nose bleeds with general inflammation of nasal passages and often other related areas such as mouth and throat.

Ipecac – spasmodic, intermittent bleeding and bright red blood. Often accompanied by bouts of coughing and occasional vomiting.

Lachesis – dark blood from nose, purplish or almost black in color. Often a result of severe infections in throat, sinuses, and nasal passages.

OTHER

An **ice pack** and pressure on the nose will help to stop a major nose bleed.

Pneumonia and bronchitis

Bronchitis is an inflammation or infection of the airways leading from the windpipe into the lungs; pneumonia is an inflammation or infection of the lung tissue.

The symptoms: are persistent coughing and chest discomfort; lethargy and poor appetite; and perhaps a nasal discharge. Breathing can be rapid or difficult and sometimes there is a high temperature.

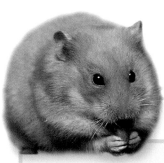

Hamsters are especially prone to pneumonia.

The causes are quite varied:
- Infections – viral, bacterial, or fungal.
- Allergies – acute reactions to allergens such as pollens will cause bronchitis.
- Parasites – lungworm, but also the larvae of ordinary roundworms, which migrate through lung tissue on a journey round the body, causing an inflammatory reaction.
- Foreign bodies – inhaling undesirable material, such as food particles, grass seeds, small household articles. Also dusts, smoke, and other irritants.
- Chinchillas are especially prone to pneumonia if their housing is damp or draughty.
- Pneumonia in hamsters is the second most common disease – after diarrhea.

CAUSES

- infection
- allergy
- parasites
- foreign bodies

SIGNS AND SYMPTOMS

- persistent cough
- chest discomfort
- nasal discharge
- breathing may be rapid or difficult
- high temperature

REMEDIES

Any necessary veterinary treatment for pneumonia or bronchitis will be enhanced by the following medicines:

AROMATHERAPY
Hyssop – for severe coughing, and pneumonia following a spread of infection from the upper respiratory tract, such as kennel cough or cat influenza.
Lavender – for bronchitis and pneumonia following throat infection, especially where the patient has bad breath. Often the pneumonia follows a period of stress or anxiety – such as after a move of home, or the introduction of a new pet into the household.
Tea tree – a powerful antiseptic and anti-infective remedy in pneumonia and bronchitis.
Peppermint – bronchitis with a spasmodic cough, and sometimes asthmatic symptoms.
Eucalyptus – catarrhal bronchitis, congested lungs, often following throat infections or tonsillitis.

HERBAL
Garlic – the great respiratory purifier. It clears lungs, helping to remove mucus from them. Anti-infective too.

HOMEOPATHY
Belladonna – patient is feverish, pupils often dilated. There is intermittent coughing, and the chest is painful. The patient feels hot, and may be very tender when touched.
Hepar sulph. – for infective pneumonia, where there is a infected discharge from the nostrils.
Kreosotum – in acute infective pneumonias, with hemorrhages in and under the skin as well as hemorrhage in the form of nose bleeds.
Ant. tart. – much wheezing and congestion. Mucus on the lungs, but little is coughed up.
Bryonia – pneumonia and bronchitis where the symptoms are worse when the patient gets up and moves, but are better for rest and quiet. Patient often lies on the affected side of the chest, since symptoms are relieved by pressure.
Drosera – violent coughing; pneumonia usually caused by virus infections.
Lycopodium – difficult breathing and a fan-like movement in the nostrils, leading to acute pneumonia.
Phosphorus – pneumonia, often with a rusty-colored secretion from the lungs.

NUTRITIONAL
Vitamins C and **A** both help the body fight lung disease.

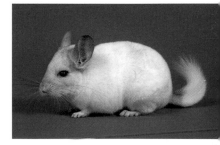

Chinchillas must be kept warm and dry to avoid pneumonia.

DOS AND DON'TS

As for sinusitis and nasal discharge (see page 92).

Lavender oil is good for bronchitis and pneumonia following throat infection.

Heart disease

CAUSES

- congenital abnormality
- endocarditis/myocarditis
- cardiomyopathy
- congestive heart disease

SIGNS AND SYMPTOMS

- coughs at night and on movement/exercise
- heart murmur
- breathlessness/panting
- lack of energy
- weight loss
- edema

Cavalier King Charles spaniels are particularly prone to heart disease, most commonly valve defects and heart murmurs.

Coronary heart disease in humans is caused mainly by furring of the arteries in the heart. However, such furring is almost unknown in pets; if it does occur, it is caused by either acquired or congenital heart defect or acute infection, rather than coronary heart disease. Most heart problems in pets are slow in onset, and there is time to diagnose and treat the condition, often successfully for long periods. Because heart surgery is rarely performed on animals, it is important to notice symptoms early and to seek treatment promptly – using conventional heart support medicines as well as natural medicines.

Small animals rarely develop heart conditions; almost all heart disease is in dogs and cats. Coughs caused by heart disease are particularly noticeable at night and on movement and exercise. The heart of a pet with severe heart problems may be so enlarged that the heartbeat can be visibly seen as a movement of the chest wall, or murmur may be distinctly heard.

- Some breeds of dogs are particularly prone to valve defects and heart murmurs – Cavalier King Charles spaniels are, unfortunately, the top breed in this respect.
- Cats are prone to cardiomyopathy, but rarely suffer other heart problems.

REMEDIES

When treating heart disease, natural medicines are compatible with the conventional drugs your veterinarian prescribes, and can often reduce the dose of drugs needed or (in some cases) remove the need for conventional drugs completely.

AROMATHERAPY
Coriander/Cilantro – a good heart support remedy, especially in old animals.
Ylang ylang – for conditions where the heart is beating too rapidly, particularly if breathing rate is rapid too. There may be high blood pressure.

FLOWER AND GEM REMEDIES
Sage is beneficial for heart disease of all kinds.

HERBAL
Cayenne – a stimulatory, invigorating herb that improves circulation and can give new life to a failing heart. Do not use for heart rhythm abnormalities, though it will help all other heart problems.
Hawthorn – tincture or infusion are a classic and effective herbal heart support treatment. Hawthorn

strengthens the heart, relaxes the arteries, and stabilizes irregular heartbeats.
Garlic – a tonic for the whole heart and circulatory system.

CRYSTAL AND GEM ESSENCES
Emerald – helps all heart problems, including rhythm abnormalities.
Jade – good for weak hearts with poor circulation.
Malachite – a heart-support remedy, especially helpful at times of stress.

HOMEOPATHY
Baryta carb. – a supportive heart remedy for the older pet.
Crataegus – a heart-strengthening remedy, especially good for valve problems and congestive heart failure.
Digitalis – for heart disease where the heart is weak and there is a slow, irregular pulse. Affected pets may have temporary black-outs or fainting

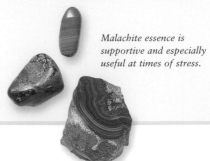

Malachite essence is supportive and especially useful at times of stress.

The symptoms are breathlessness, panting, coughing, and lack of energy, with an unwillingness to take exercise, or an inability to continue exercise – for example, a dog may need many rests while out for a walk. Additional symptoms are weight loss and edema (excess fluid in body tissues). This edema is usually noticeable first as excess fluid in the abdomen (ascites), but the legs may also become swollen.

Hawthorn will strengthen the heart and relax the arteries.

spells because insufficient oxygen reaches the brain. These are not heart attacks. Digitalis will be very effective in minimizing these black-outs.

Lycopus – for rapid, irregular heart beats, often with wheezy breathing and coughing. The patient may be thirsty and pass lots of pale urine.

Spongia tosta – especially useful for the cough that accompanies many pets affected by heart disease. Lungs are congested, and the cough is worse for exercise.

NUTRITIONAL

Taurine – some cases of cardiomyopathy in cats are associated with a taurine deficiency. Give this amino acid – or foods containing it – if necessary.

Vitamin E – helps strengthen heart muscle. Give to all pets with heart disease.

Coenzyme Q10 – another essential supplement, especially for cardiomyopathy and weakened hearts.

There are various causes:

• Congenital – pets may be born with a defective heart, as in the "hole in the heart" condition in human babies. Affected pets may not grow properly, have less energy, and be weaker than other young animals. Heart rhythm abnormalities – the nerve and electrical control of the heart is malfunctioning and the heart beats too quickly, misses beats or has erratic beats. Occasionally heart pacemakers can be fitted, but usually medicines are the main form of treatment.

• Endocarditis/myocarditis – these conditions are infections of the heart valves or heart muscle, following bacterial spread from infected wounds or infectious diseases.

• Cardiomyopathy – this is an enlargement and thickening of the heart, which may result from an overactive thyroid gland, or may develop in its own right.

• Congestive heart failure – the most common form of heart disease in pets. It is not really a disease in its own right, but is a consequence of valve defects (perhaps following endocarditis) or cardiomyopathy or myocarditis. As the heart begins to fail, fluid builds up in the body and all the classic symptoms of heart disease (see Signs and Symptoms, left) develop.

A balanced diet that is low in salt, and plenty of regular exercise will help your pet to maintain peak health and guard against heart disease.

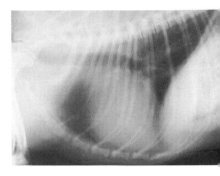

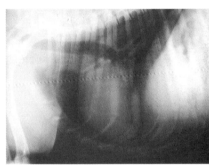

TOP *This x-ray shows a dog with an enlarged heart.*

ABOVE *This dog has a normal heart. The comparison with the x-ray above is striking.*

DOS AND DON'TS

Do use remedies for edema and congestion when these symptoms are present (see pages 98–99).

Do use remedies for shock and collapse promptly if black-outs or collapse from heart failure occur.

Do ensure diet is low in salt, and ensure pets do not become overweight – or that they lose weight if necessary.

Congestion (edema)

Edema is an excessive build-up of fluid in body tissues and is a side effect of heart and other diseases.

The symptoms are swollen, puffy legs and occasionally face, a pot-bellied appearance due to build up of fluid in abdomen (ascites), and breathing problems due to excessive fluid in lungs – usually coughing and wheezing.

Heart disease is the commonest cause of edema. However, liver conditions often cause ascites – this may be due to liver disease in its own right, or the liver may be affected as a side effect of heart disease. Also, tumors can cause edema, usually by effecting pressure on blood or lymph vessels.

Look out for symptoms of breathing difficulties and coughing in cases of edema.

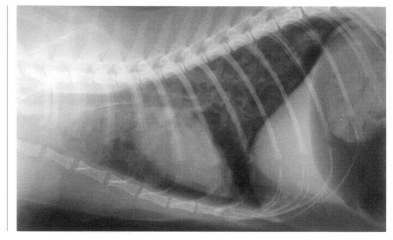

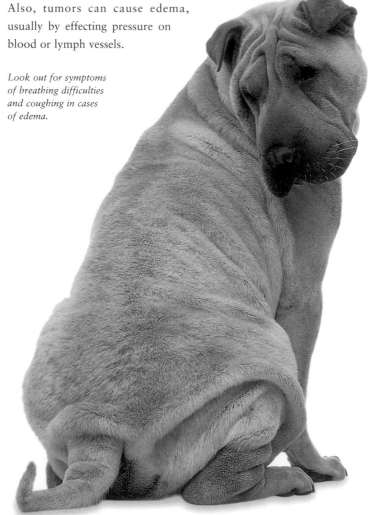

In treatment, conventional medicine usually makes use of diuretics, drugs that help to increase the amount of fluid passed out by the body. Natural medicines are often a more gentle way of balancing the body's fluid input and output. They can be given to pets already on diuretics as an extra support, or even as a replacement.

AROMATHERAPY
Coriander/Cilantro – a excellent natural diuretic aid, especially for weak, debilitated pets.
Cypress – good for lung congestion, generally poor circulation, and for anxious pets.
Fennel – a circulatory support; for poor appetite.
Ginger – stimulates circulation and a general tonic for lethargic pets.
Lime and lemon – both good for congestion, in circulation or in sinuses.
Rosemary – for fluid retention, caused by either heart or liver disease.

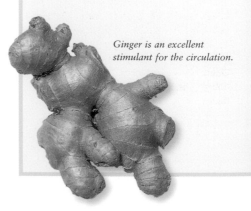

Ginger is an excellent stimulant for the circulation.

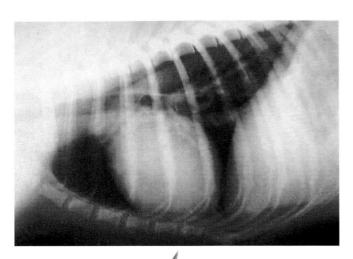

FAR LEFT *This cat is suffering from a build-up of fluid in the lungs, which can be seen here as a gray shadow.*

LEFT *This dog has a healthy lung – the organ can clearly be seen and the chest cavity is clear of fluid.*

CAUSES

- heart disease
- liver conditions
- tumor

SIGNS AND SYMPTOMS

- swollen puffy legs/face
- pot-bellied appearance
- breathing problems
- coughing and wheezing

REMEDIES

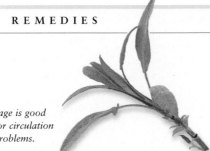

Sage is good for circulation problems.

Sandalwood – especially good for respiratory congestion since it opens up the airways.
White thyme – for general poor circulation, especially if muscle and joint problems are present.

FLOWER AND GEM REMEDIES
Sage helps reduce symptoms of all circulatory problems, including congestion.

HERBAL
Cayenne – stimulates circulation and relieves congestion.
Dandelion – a superb natural diuretic, whether fluid retention is caused by heart problems or liver disease. Often given in combination with other greenleaf herbs, such as **parsley** and **nettles**.
Elderberry – a good diuretic and blood purifier.
Ginkgo – improves circulation and blood supply to all tissues.
Parsley – another natural herbal diuretic.

CRYSTAL AND GEM ESSENCES
Agate – Brown agate is used for fluid retention.
Bloodstone – for all blood disorders, including congestion.
Emerald – for edema associated with heart disease.

HOMEOPATHY
Apis mel. – for swollen tissues, especially if they pit (leave a depression for a short time after being pressed with finger).
Crataegus – for congestive heart failure, helps both heart and circulation.
Eel serum – a natural homeopathic diuretic, especially if kidney problems are also present.
Secale – improves circulation to damaged tissue, so will help to relieve the swelling that can occur at the site of damage.

NUTRITIONAL
Potassium – if conventional diuretics are being used, excessive amounts of potassium may be lost with the fluid. A potassium supplement is advisable (your veterinarian will advise on dosage if this is necessary).

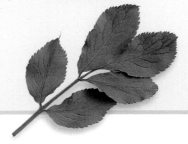

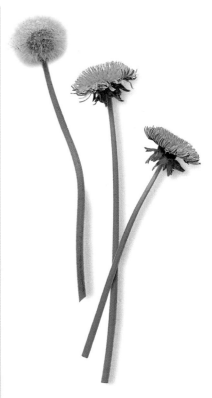

ABOVE *Dandelion is a very effective natural diuretic.*

LEFT *Elderberry is a natural diuretic and blood purifier.*

Anemia

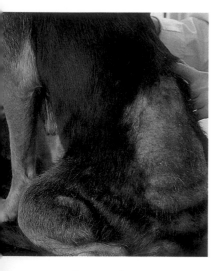

Parasite infestation may be a cause of anemia.

Anemia is a deficiency of circulating red blood cells in the bloodstream. An anemic pet will have pale lips, gums, and conjunctive, and be weak and tired.

The various causes include:

• Hemorrhage – blood loss after accidents and injuries, or after poisoning.

• Parasites – both blood-sucking parasites, such as fleas and lice, or parasites in the blood itself.

• Feline infectious anemia.

• Infections – can damage red blood cells leading to anemia.

• Clotting defects – conditions where the blood does not clot properly, leading to excessive blood loss. These defects may be genetic, or caused by toxins in the blood.

• Bleeding disorders – these are mainly genetic defects affecting the ability of the blood to maintain normal function, and to clot normally.

• Auto-immune disease – the immune system mistakenly recognizes the body's own blood cells as foreign tissue and destroys them.

• Dietary deficiencies – a lack of vitamins B12 and C, and the minerals copper, cobalt, and iron can all cause anemia.

• Kidney disease – may affect the kidneys ability to secrete a hormone called erythro-poetin, needed for normal red blood cell production, and this can lead to anemia.

• Bone marrow disease – red blood cells are produced from the bone marrow, so any disease affecting marrow, such as feline leukemia virus, is likely to cause anemia.

REMEDIES

In treating anemia, blood transfusions may be required in an emergency. Any causes such as parasites or poison should be removed. There are many good supporting remedies for pets with anemia.

AROMATHERAPY
Angelica root – for anemia, especially in tense, nervous individuals.
Marjoram – particularly helps blood loss and anemia in females with reproductive problems, and is a general strengthening remedy.

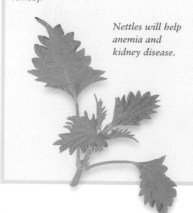

Nettles will help anemia and kidney disease.

FLOWER AND GEM REMEDIES
Hornbeam – an excellent strengthening remedy for weak, anemic pets.
Ruby – helps to restore normal coloring.

HERBAL
Elderberry – for all blood disorders, including anemia.
Nettles – for anemia, especially where kidney disease is present.
Kelp – the minerals, vitamins, and trace elements in kelp are useful for anemia, especially if there is a dietary deficiency.

CRYSTAL AND GEM ESSENCES
Ruby – for anemia of all kinds.

HOMEOPATHY
Ferrum net. – ideal for anemia, especially if poor nutrition is a factor.
Natrum mur. – weakness and anemia, especially where kidney disease is present.
China – for anemia with great weakness.
Cuprum met. – where insufficient red blood cells are being produced.

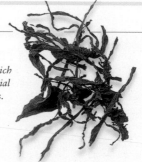

Kelp is rich in essential nutrients.

Crotalus horridus – where Warfarin poisoning is the cause.
Lachesis – for clotting disorders with dark, purple hemorrhage.
Phosphorus – for persistent bleeding of bright red blood.
Secale – where there are multiple hemorrhages under the skin.

NUTRITIONAL
Iron, B vitamins, vitamin C, and any minerals missing from the diet should be given as a supplement.
Vitamin K is a specific antidote to Warfarin poison (usually given by injection at the start of treatment).

Thrombosis

Thrombosis is the formation of a blood clot inside a blood vessel, blocking the flow of blood to body tissues.

The symptoms are pain and discomfort in the area beyond the thrombosis (blood clot). If a large area of the body loses blood supply, shock and gangrene may set in.

This condition can be caused by heart or circulatory disease – all types affect the usual flow of blood. Surgery can bring it on – recovery is complicated by post-operative thrombosis occuring in the lungs after the (necessary) trauma of surgery.

The commonest form of thrombosis is iliac, or aortic, thrombosis of cats. In this condition, a blood clot forms at the point where the aorta (the main blood vessel for the heart) divides to supply the hind legs.

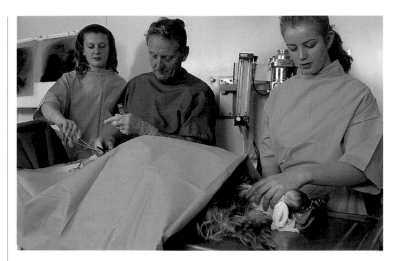

Affected cats suddenly lose the use of their hind legs, which become cold to the touch. This condition is extremely painful, and cats may collapse and go into shock.

ABOVE *Thrombosis can occur in the lungs as a post-operative complication.*

LEFT *To relieve shock, Aconite may be given immediately following collapse from thrombosis.*

REMEDIES

Thrombosis is always potentially life-threatening and immediate veterinary treatment is necessary. Natural medicines can help the collapse and shock, and minimize the damage caused by the lack of circulation to the affected area.

FLOWER AND GEM REMEDIES
Bach Rescue Remedy for the shock and circulatory deficiency.

Yarrow will have the action of helping a blood clot to dissolve slowly.

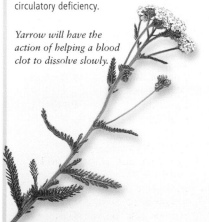

AROMATHERAPY
Lavender and **vervain** – calming and soothing agents.
Yarrow – specific for thrombosis; will help the blood clot to dissolve slowly.

HOMEOPATHY
Aconite – for the shock; can be alternated with doses of Rescue Remedy.
Veratrum alb. – for collapse, with coldness of affected part.
Secale – because the effect of secale is to improve circulation to tissues deprived of normal blood supply, it is the ideal remedy to use to aid recovery after thrombosis. It will help prevent gangrene developing, and may avoid complications, or even euthanasia, which is often the tragic consequence of thrombosis.
Opium – will help the weakness and paralysis that often follows thrombosis.

CAUSES

- heart or circulatory disease
- surgery

SIGNS AND SYMPTOMS

- pain and discomfort in area beyond blood clot
- loss of feeling in the limbs
- swelling (again often in the limbs)
- shock
- gangrene

Hypothyroidism

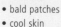

CAUSES

- may be unknown
- pituitary disease may be involved
- may be a form of auto-immune disease

SIGNS AND SYMPTOMS

- increasing body weight
- loss of energy
- poor condition of skin and coat
- bald patches
- cool skin

Underactive thyroid glands are a common medical condition in dogs, but overactive thyroids are rare. This is the exact reverse of the situation in cats.

The symptoms are increasing body weight, loss of energy, and poor condition of skin and coat, with coarse, harsh fur. There may be bald patches, with the pattern of baldness the same on both sides of the body. Fur is often lost first on the flanks. The heart rate slows down, so the patient feels the cold and needs to be much warmer than usual. Unneutered females will stop having seasons, unneutered males will lose their libido. The loss of energy can be quite marked – no desire to go for walks, sleeping much more than usual. Appetite may increase, but bodyweight increases even if the affected pet is not eating more than usual. The skin may feel cool to the touch, and is not itchy.

The causes are often not known. Pituitary disease can be involved. It is now thought that many thyroid problems may be a form of auto-immune disease – the body begins to recognize the thyroid tissue as foreign and destroys it.

Most smaller pets do not suffer from underactive thyroids, but budgerigars do sometimes show symptoms if their diet is deficient in iodine. One of the most noticeable symptoms in budgies is that they begin to make a high-pitched noise, rather like a squeaking wheel that needs oiling.

REMEDIES

For treatment, conventional thyroid hormone supplements may be needed, but the following natural remedies may mean they are not necessary, or can be given in a reduced dose.

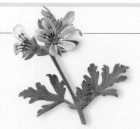

Geranium stimulates the hormone system.

AROMATHERAPY
Clary sage – a hormone-balancing essential oil, both for female hormonal problems but also for thyroid imbalances.
Geranium – a stimulant to the hormonal system, both for the adrenal glands and the thyroid.

FLOWER AND GEM REMEDIES
Topaz is a hormone-balancing gem remedy for under- and overactive thyroids.
Hornbeam and **olive** help improve energy levels.

HERBAL
Kelp is high in iodine and other minerals needed to maintain the thyroid glands in good working order. It is derived from seaweed.

An underactive thyroid can cause increased weight.

Garlic is also high in iodine, and helps regulate thyroid function.

CRYSTAL AND GEM ESSENCES
Chrysocolla, peridot, sodalite, and **tiger's eye** are all crystals that regulate and balance thyroid gland function.

Tiger's eye is useful to regulate and balance thyroid function.

HOMEOPATHY
Thyroidinum – good for the skin symptoms of hypothyroidism, although it is more helpful for overactive thyroids in most instances.
Calc. carb. – a useful remedy for hypothyroidism. Suits slow, overweight animals needing warmth.
Iris vers. – has a stimulating effect on many glands, including the thyroid.

Hyperthyroidism

Overactive thyroid glands are a problem seen mainly in cats. The symptoms are an increase in thirst and appetite, but a marked weight loss. There is also diarrhea and sometimes vomiting, along with weakness and loss of muscle strength in particular. Restlessness is common, despite the weakness. Heart and breathing rates increase.

It can be caused by tumors or natural hypertrophy (increase in size and thickness) of the thyroid glands.

Cats are notorious for developing kidney problems as they age, the symptoms of which are similar to hyperthyroidism (weight loss, increased thirst, and so on). Blood tests may be needed to ascertain which problem – or if both – is present.

CAUSES

- tumor
- hypertrophy of the thyroid glands

SIGNS AND SYMPTOMS

- increase in thirst and appetite
- marked weight loss
- diarrhea
- vomiting
- weakness/loss of muscle strength
- restlessness
- increase in heart and breathing rates

REMEDIES

Conventional treatment involves the use of drugs, surgery to remove one or both thyroid glands, or the use of radioactive iodine to kill off excess thyroid tissue. Natural medicines can often mean these treatments are not necessary, or that lower doses of drugs can be given.

Clary sage is an essential oil that will balance hormones and improve thyroid function.

AROMATHERAPY
Clary sage – to balance hormones; can help return thyroid function to normal.

FLOWER AND GEM REMEDIES
Topaz helps both under- and overactive glands to become stable.
Impatiens reduces the irritability and restlessness.

HERBAL
Bugleweed infusion will help treat symptoms of hyperthyroidism.

CRYSTAL AND GEM ESSENCES
Chrysocolla, peridot, sodalite, and **tiger's eye** all stabilize thyroid activity.

HOMEOPATHY
Iodum – suits the typical hyperthyroid symptoms of ravenous appetite, loss of weight, restlessness, and weakness. Urine may be dark and strong-smelling. The skin is often dry and leathery.
Natrum mur. – greatly increased thirst, weakness of legs, dry or greasy skin, and loss of bodily condition.
Thyroidinum – anemia, emaciation, and muscular weakness, together with an increase in heart rate.

Lycopus – will help with the rapid heart rate and reduce the likelihood of permanent heart damage.

All hormonal problems are likely to be triggered or aggravated by stress and emotional traumas. Ensure the pet's environment is as stress-free as possible, and give stress-relieving remedies if appropriate.

Overactive thyroid glands are more common in cats, causing increased appetite and thirst.

Diabetes mellitus and insipidus

CAUSES

- injury or tumor of the pancreas
- side-effect of steroids
- may be unknown

SIGNS AND SYMPTOMS

- greatly increased thirst and appetite
- increased volume of urine passed
- weight loss
- cataracts
- vomiting
- dullness and depression

ENDOCRINE SYSTEM

Hypothyroidism, Hyperthyroidism, Diabetes mellitus and insipidus, Cushing's disease, Addison's disease, Hypokalemia – All these conditions relate to the network of glands that secrete the hormones which control many body processes and metabolism. The most important glands in this system are the thyroid glands, the pituitary glands in the brain, the adrenal glands, and areas of the pancreas that produce insulin.

The thyroid glands can malfunction by being overactive or underactive. Too little thyroid activity is known as hypothyroidism; excessive thyroid activity is called hyperthyroidism.

There are two forms of diabetes and each should be addressed as a separate problem. Diabetes mellitus is commonly known as "sugar diabetes." Diabetes insipidus is a malfunction in the fluid balance control system of the body.

DIABETES MELLITUS

In the case of diabetes mellitus, there is a lack of sufficient insulin hormone in the bloodstream to enable glucose to be transported from the blood into the body cells. Glucose is the body's main energy source, and without proper absorption, serious life-threatening symptoms soon develop.

These are: greatly increased thirst and appetite; increased volume of urine passed; weight loss; liver enlargement; sudden, rapid onset of cataracts; vomiting; a dull and depressed patient.

It can be caused by injury or tumor of the pancreas or as a side-effect of long-term administration of steroids or female hormones. Sometimes the cause is unknown.

Diabetes can occur in most mammals, but among pets is seen regularly only in dogs and cats. If you suspect your pet has

TESTING FOR DIABETES

Diabetes mellitus causes sugar (glucose) to be passed in the urine. This can be tested by a simple "dipstick" test with a strip containing an agent that changes color on the presence of sugar. Diabetes insipidus causes a change in the specific gravity of the urine. This is tested in a similar way.

Both forms of diabetes can be diagnosed from urine analysis.

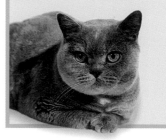

diabetes, take a urine sample to your veterinarian for analysis.

DIABETES INSIPIDUS

In the case of diabetes insipidus, there is a failure in the control of water balance within the body.

REMEDIES FOR DIABETES INSIPIDUS

Conventional treatment is usually the administration of extracts of the pituitary gland, which contains ADH, but results are variable. Natural remedies are often effective in controlling symptoms.

FLOWER AND GEM REMEDIES
Topaz helps balance any hormone dysfunction, including diabetes insipidus.

Topaz balances hormone function.

CRYSTAL AND GEM ESSENCES
Chrysocolla, **peridot**, **sodalite**, and **tiger's eye** also stabilize hormone imbalance, and all of them are calming, soothing stones, which help deal with the tendency to be restless and anxious when affected by diabetes insipidus.

HOMEOPATHY
Uranium nit. – an effective remedy for diabetes insipidus.
Iris vers. – can be used in the treatment of both diabetes mellitis and insipidus.

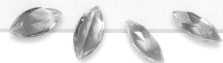

REMEDIES FOR DIBETES MELLITUS

Treating diabetes in pets almost always requires the use of insulin injections. If treated in the early stages, natura medicines can sometimes be sufficient. If not, the use of natural remedies often means that lower doses of insulin are required.

FLOWER AND GEM REMEDIES
Topaz is a balancing agent for all hormonal problems.
Sugar beet is an excellent flower remedy to help control diabetes.
Hornbeam and **olive** are strengthening and alleviate lethargy and weakness.

HERBAL

Onions and **garlic** lower blood-sugar levels.

Garlic will slowly but effectively lower blood sugar.

Although slow in acting (compared to insulin), they are effective, and should be taken regularly by diabetic pets. Because a few instances of onion poisoning have been recorded, it is important to give small but regular amounts.
Fenugreek seeds – a decoction of fenugreek, or proprietary tablets containing fenugreek, will also help to control diabetes.
Oak bark, olive root, and **Great Northern/haricot bean pods** all have an action in reducing sugar levels.

CRYSTAL AND GEM ESSENCES
Chrysocolla, peridot, sodalite, and **tiger's eye** all help stabilize levels of hormones, including insulin.

HOMEOPATHY
Iris vers. – helps pancreatic problems of all kinds, including diabetes.

Onion can be given in regular small doses.

Syzygium – an excellent remedy to to maintain lower sugar levels.
Acid phos. – for the weakness and debility of diabetes.
Uranium nit. – reduces sugar levels, reduces thirst and urine output.

NUTRITIONAL
A **low-sugar diet** is important. Luckily, most pet diets do not normally contain many sugars – but check the ingredients of your pet food carefully. It is equally important when insulin treatment is being given to feed a single, standard diet, with no variation, and at exact set intervals. Even if insulin treatment is not being administered, set meals of fixed volume are best – the body's insulin levels will vary less.

The symptoms are greatly increased thirst, and increased output of pale, weak urine.

Common causes include kidney disease, which prevents the kidney from responding to the hormone that controls water balance (ADH), and failure of ADH production, because of pituitary gland damage caused by injuries from tumors. Diabetes insipidus is seen mainly in dogs.

Diagnosing the condition can be difficult, and complicated measurements of precise fluid intake and output may be necessary in order to make a positive diagnosis of diabetes insipidus.

CAUSES

- kidney disease
- failure of ADH production

SIGNS AND SYMPTOMS

- greatly increased thirst
- increased output of pale, weak urine

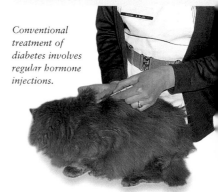

Conventional treatment of diabetes involves regular hormone injections.

DOS AND DON'TS

Do remember both forms of diabetes are serious conditions – do not treat them with natural remedies only, unless advised to do so by your veterinarian.

Do try to remember the earliest signs of both forms of diabetes. There may have been a trigger to the symptoms – which can possibly be removed or treated even now.

Do remind your veterinarian that your pet is diabetic if any new drugs are given. Some drugs (such as steroids) are potentially dangerous to give a diabetic pet.

Do remember that pets can be accidently overdosed with insulin – have something sweet and sugary ready should a diabetic coma begin to occur.

Do remember stress and emotional trauma can aggravate symptoms of diabetes – give your pet a stress-free life, if possible.

Do be careful when unneutered bitches or cats come in season. This can rapidly upset a controlled diabetic state. Neutering may need to be carried out to prevent this destabilization.

Cushing's disease and Addison's disease

CAUSES

- pituitary gland disease
- adrenal gland disease
- injury
- tumor
- auto-immune disease
- side-effects of drugs

SIGNS AND SYMPTOMS

- increased thirst and appetite
- increases volume of urine passed
- muscle wasting/weakness
- liver-enlargement
- bald patches
- thinning of skin

DOS AND DON'TS – CUSHINGS

Do remember to tell any new veterinarian who treats your pet that Cushing's has been diagnosed. If some drugs including steroids were administered, they could aggravate symptoms.

Do start your pet on a supplementation program such as vitamins C and B-complex.

ADDISON'S

Do have steroids available for immediate administration should a sudden deterioration occur.

Do remember that at times of stress an Addisonian crisis could be triggered. Be prepared.

The adrenal glands are the production site for the body's natural steroids. If production goes wrong and too few or too many steroids are produced, major problems ensue. The main diseases of the adrenals are Cushing's disease and Addison's disease.

CUSHING'S DISEASE

Cushing's disease is an overproduction of glucocortoids from the adrenal glands.

The symptoms are: increased thirst and hunger; increased urine; muscle wasting and weakness – often seen as a drooping belly; liver enlargement; symmetrical bald patches; thinning skin and formation of small hard calcium deposits in the skin.

It is caused by disease of the pituitary gland, which secretes a controlling hormone, ACTH, that stimulates production of steroids by the adrenals. If ACTH levels rise, the adrenals will produce more steroids. Other causes include adrenal gland disease – injury, tumors, or auto-immune disease. It can also be drug-induced – overuse of steroids will induce signs of Cushing's.

The disease is seen mainly in dogs, though it can occur in other species (horses are prone to Cushing's disease).

REMEDIES

Only one drug is available to treat Cushing's, and it is potentially highly toxic; great care needs to be taken over its use. Surgery on the pituitary gland is occasionally undertaken, but results are variable. Natural medicines have a good record of treating Cushing's.

ACUPUNCTURE
Often used in combination with natural medicines as a treatment for Cushing's.

FLOWER AND GEM REMEDIES
Olive and **hornbeam** help energize the debilitated Cushing's patient.

HERBAL
Garlic helps balance steroid production and reduce excessive levels.
Dandelion, **nettles**, **watercress**, and **parsley** also help to stabilize the symptoms.

HOMEOPATHY
Following the principle of homeopathy – a minute, potentized dose of a substance that causes symptoms will cure those same symptoms – these remedies will naturally treat Cushing's:
Cortisone and **ACTH** – it is possible in homeopathy to make a remedy from these hormones and use them as (very successful) treatments.

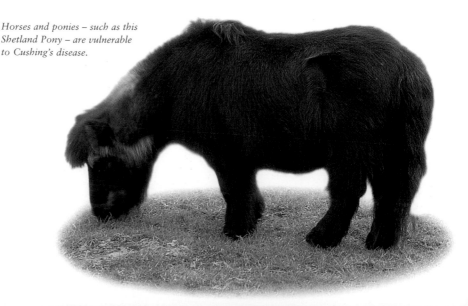

Horses and ponies – such as this Shetland Pony – are vulnerable to Cushing's disease.

Hypokalemia

ADDISON'S DISEASE

Addison's disease is also termed hypoadrenocorticism and is an under-production of steroids by the adrenals.

The symptoms are: vomiting and diarrhea; muscular weakness and trembling; weight loss; weak pulse and dehydration, slow heart rate; increased thirst and increased output of urine. In later stages, collapse and shock occur. Not all symptoms may develop, and in the early stages the signs may be difficult to diagnose.

Addison's is mainly seen in dogs, but sometimes occurs in other species. Diagnosis depends on blood tests, which are quite complicated to perform.

It can be caused by injuries, tumors, and thrombosis, or from overuse of mitotane. This drug, which treats Cushing's, will bring on symptoms of Addison's. Sudden cessation of long-term steroids will induce symptoms of Addison's. Steroids should always be withdrawn very slowly.

REMEDIES

Conventional treatment is long-term steroids. Natural remedies can successfully reduce, and in some cases remove, the need for steroids.

AROMATHERAPY
Rosemary, **ginger**, and **lemongrass** will strengthen adrenals and steroid production

FLOWER AND GEM REMEDIES
Olive and **hornbeam** are strengthening and stimulating.

HERBAL
Dandelion, **parsley**, **watercress**, and **nettle** all help to balance steroid production.

HOMEOPATHY
Natrum mur. – helps treat some symptoms of Addison's, such as weakness and thirst.

This is a low potassium level in the bloodstream. Although not strictly an endocrine problem since it is not caused by a hormone imbalance or one of the endocrine glands, it is a metabolic imbalance, which is why it is included in this section.

The symptoms are muscle weakness leading to difficult breathing; weight loss, lethargy, and anemia; poor appetite; poor coat condition.

The causes can be a side-effect of chronic kidney disease or of diabetes mellitus; gastroenteritis, leading to potassium loss because of diarrhea; dietary (insufficient potassium in diet), not necessarily because the diet is low in potassium, but because potassium is being lost from the body.

REMEDIES

Hypokalemia is a problem seen almost solely in cats. Treat it in the following ways:

NUTRITIONAL
Potassium supplementation – potassium, in a powder form that can be added to the diet, is available. Bananas are rich in potassium.

FLOWER AND GEM REMEDIES
Olive and **hornbeam** will strengthen animals weakened by hypokalaemia.

HOMOEOPATHY
Kali chlor. – will help, especially where the symptoms are a consequence of kidney disease.
Kali carb. – ideal for the weaker, older animal.

CRYSTAL AND GEM ESSENCES
Ruby will support and strengthen cats with hypokalemia.

CAUSES

- side-effect of chronic kidney disease or diabetes mellitus
- gastroenteritis
- dietary

SIGNS AND SYMPTOMS

- muscle weakness
- weight loss
- lethargy
- anemia
- poor appetite
- poor coat condition

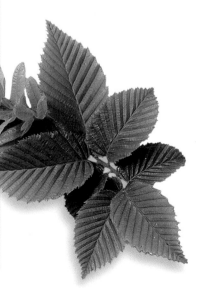

Hornbeam will strengthen weakness from hypokalemia.

Musculoskeletal disorders

CAUSES

- accidents and injuries
- infection
- immune system disease
- natural deterioration of age
- inappropriate exercise
- dietary and metabolic causes
- congenital conditions

SIGNS AND SYMPTOMS

- pale lips and gums
- tired weakness

RIGHT *The fractured tibia bone of a young puppy.*

FAR RIGHT *The tibia bone of the same puppy – now being repaired with a metal pin.*

This system consists of the muscles, joints, tendons, ligaments, and bones of the body. Specific natural medicines for the different conditions will follow. However, the therapies below will help relieve pain and aid recovery in all of the conditions listed on pages 108–120. They should always be considered along with the other remedies listed.

Disorders of the musculoskeletal system usually cause one or more of the following symptoms: lameness and stiffness; overall weakness; clear pain on movement and unwillingness to exercise (your dog may resist from its usual daily walk).

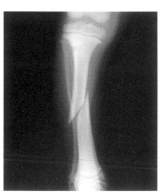
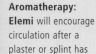
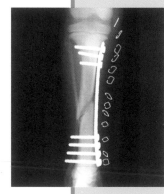

BONE FRACTURES

All fractures of bones will need help rapid attention from your veterinarian. This may in the form of a splint or a plaster, or in the case of serious fractures will need surgery and the use of metal pins, plates, screws, or wires. Natural remedies can speed up the rate of healing of fractured bones.

Homeopathy: Symphytum accelerates bone healing in all cases. **Calc. carb.** increases healing rates in heavily built, overweight pets.

Herbs: Aloe vera gel, applied externally, will help healing. **Comfrey root** – small amounts by mouth, is ideal (it's common name is Boneknit).

Aromatherapy: Elemi will encourage circulation after a plaster or splint has been removed

Nutritional therapy: Give extra **calcium, magnesium, boron,** and **phosphorus** to facilitate bone strengthening.

Massage is not only an effective treatment for stiff and painful joints and muscles but will also be enjoyed by your pet.

THERAPIES

ACUPUNCTURE
Especially good for pain relief and both to stimulate healing and slow down deterioration of joints.

MASSAGE
Particularly for stiff and painful joints and muscles.

OSTEOPATHY AND CHIROPRACTIC
Especially for spinal problems.

PHYSIOTHERAPY
Particularly for accelerating recovery after injuries.

MAGNETIC THERAPY
Good for pain relief and to prevent deterioration in joint disease.

Arthritis

The inflamed joints symptomatic of arthritis are one of the commonest conditions of older pets.

The symptoms include pain and stiffness in one or more joints. The joint may be hot and swollen, or simply stiff. There may be atrophy (shrinking) of muscles around the joint from lack of use.

It is caused by wear and tear – simple deterioration of old age is the most frequent cause. This may be exacerbated by poor confirmation (shape and position) of joints

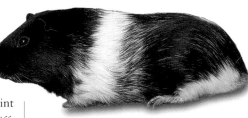

A diet deficient in Vitamin C can cause painful swollen joints in guinea pigs.

– such as in hip dysplasia. It can also arise from injuries and infections and from immune system disease – some arthritic damage is the result of the body mistakenly recognizing the joint tissue as foreign and destroying it. A poor imbalanced diet can let arthritis develop.

All species of animal can develop arthritis (except fish). The condition is most common in dogs.

- Guinea pigs may suffer swollen painful joints as a result of vitamin C deficiency – always ensure guinea pigs have sufficient vitamin C in their diet.
- Birds with arthritis may have problems in gripping their perches, and tend to fall off easily.

CAUSES

- aging
- poor shape and position of joints
- injury
- poor diet
- infection
- immune system disease

SIGNS AND SYMPTOMS

- pain and stiffness in one or more joints
- shrinking of muscles around joint

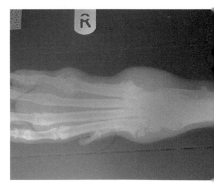

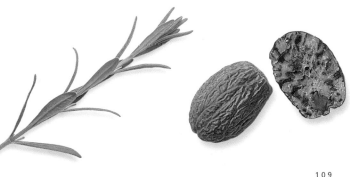

LEFT *As older dogs become stiff with arthritis, it is helpful to assist with their mobility.*

BELOW LEFT *Lavender oil is helpful in treating arthritis and is safe to apply as a massage oil.*

ABOVE *This x-ray shows inflammation around joints – symptomatic of stage two arthritis.*

BELOW RIGHT *Nutmeg improves the blood supply to the joints and slows deterioration.*

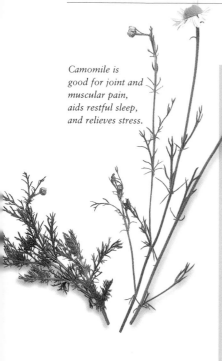

Camomile is good for joint and muscular pain, aids restful sleep, and relieves stress.

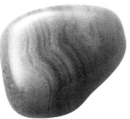

ABOVE *Blue lace agate relieves pain, stiffness, and lameness.*

BELOW *Feverfew is a natural painkiller and especially relieves hot swollen joints.*

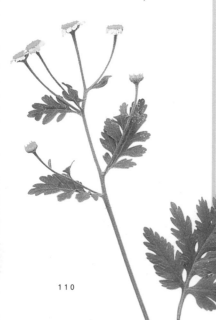

REMEDIES

Conventional treatment involves the use of anti-inflammatory agents and painkillers, either non-steroidal (preferably) or steroidal. These only palliate symptoms and do not prevent deterioration. Many drugs have side-effects if used for long periods. Natural medicines are both effective at relieving symptoms, and at helping slow down or prevent joint deterioration.

AROMATHERAPY
Gentle massage with diluted essential oils is an ideal treatment for arthritis. Many oils are beneficial, especially:

Camphor – for inflamed joints, and aches and pains in muscles and joints generally.
Camomile (German and Roman) – reduces inflammation in joints.
Juniper – helps remove toxins from damaged joints.
Lavender – a soothing, relaxing, and anti-inflammatory oil.
Marjoram – relieves stiffness in joints and improves overall mobility.
Nutmeg – improves blood supply to joints, helping to prevent deterioration.
Parsley seed – removes accumulation of toxins from joints, stimulates healing.
Pine needle – good for improving mobility and reducing discomfort.
Thyme – for all joint conditions; reduces stiffness and pain.
Yarrow – an effective natural anti-inflammatory agent.

FLOWER AND GEM REMEDIES
Crab apple – a natural cleanser and detoxifier for arthritic patients.
Ruby – a natural anti-arthritic essence; soothes aching joints.
Dill – for joints with bony lumps and spurs.

HERBAL
Yarrow – a classic herbal anti-arthritic, for the aches and pains of stiff joints.
Burdock – a detoxifier, good to use in combination with specific anti-arthritic herbs, such as yarrow, to enhance the effect.
Devil's claw – a well known anti-inflammatory herb, for joint problems of all kinds, especially arthritic hips and spine.
Nettles – something that causes a stinging pain can be used to relieve the pain and inflammation of arthritis.
Parsley – one of the so-called greenleaf herbs, it is ideal to use in combination with other herbs, such as nettles, dandelion, and watercress to treat arthritis.
White willow – the bark of the white willow contains natural aspirin-like compounds, and so is ideal for the pain and discomfort of arthritis.
Feverfew – a natural painkiller, especially good for the hot, painful, swollen joints and for back pain.

CRYSTAL AND GEM ESSENCES
Blue lace agate – an ideal crystal for arthritic pets to wear, it relieves pain, stiffness, and lameness.
Glaciated copper – effective for swollen joints and spinal arthritis.
Rutilated quartz – a pain-relieving crystal, especially for back pain.

HOMEOPATHY
Of the thousands of homeopathic remedies, dozens will help arthritis. The most important for arthritis in pets are:
Acid sal. – for stiffness and pain in small joints (toes, wrists, and ankles).
Apis mel. – for hot, shiny, swollen, sensitive joints.
Arnica – not always thought of as an arthritic remedy. As it helps heal any damaged, traumatized body tissue, it will help heal the damaged tissue within an arthritic joint. Often combined with Rhus tox. and Ruta grav. to provide an all-round effective arthritis treatment.
Belladonna – for hot and very painful joints, after injury or infection in particular.
Bryonia – for dry, stiff joints that often make a cracking noise on movement. The pain and stiffness is better at rest, worse for movement.
Calc. carb. – for arthritic pets that are slow, overweight, lazy, and love warmth.
Causticum – for stiffness with tearing pains in joints obviously painful to flex and extend. Suits old, semi-senile pets. Usually symptoms are better in warm, damp weather.
Caulophyllum – for arthritis of knees, hock, and other small joints.
Hecla lava – for bony lumps and growths on bones and joints (especially good for bone tumors).
Pulsatilla – for arthritis where symptoms shift from joint to joint. One day a knee is stiff, next day a shoulder, and so on.

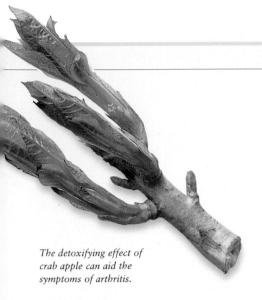

The detoxifying effect of crab apple can aid the symptoms of arthritis.

Rhus tox. – probably the best known homeopathic anti-arthritic, where stiffness is worst at rest, and the affected pet can't get comfortable. First movement on getting up is very stiff and painful, then the stiffness improves with continued movement. Symptoms are worse in cold, damp weather. Better in warm, dry weather.

NUTRITIONAL

Cider vinegar – in drinking water (1 teaspoon per 2½ cups/1 pint) is a good long-term anti-arthritic remedy.

Vitamin C – needed for healthy bones and joints. A supplement should be given to all pets with arthritis.

Vitamins A, C, and **E**, plus **selenium** (mineral) – a good detoxifying combination to cleanse and purify diseased joints.

Cod liver oil – a natural lubricant. Fish oils contain fatty acids, which are synthesized in the body into natural anti-inflammatory agents that particularly help prevent deterioration of joints. Apart from cod liver oil, halibut, salmon, and herring oils are effective anti-inflammatories. Fish oil combined with evening primrose oil or borage oil is an even better anti-inflammatory mixture, both for eczema and for arthritis. Overdose of fish oils can occur with prolonged use, particularly in cats. Consult your veterinarian about dosage if in doubt.

Magnesium – this mineral is required to form synovial fluid, the fluid which lubricates joints. In dry, cracking, stiff joints, a magnesium supplement will be beneficial.

Perna mussel – regular supplementation with perna mussel will slow down deterioration of joints, and can reverse damage in many cases, leading to greater mobility and use of joints.

Glycosaminoglycans – all nutritional supplements containing these natural joint-repairing agents will help arthritis symptoms. Perna mussel, cartilage products (shark and bovine), and chondroitin supplements are all effective in the treatment of arthritis.

Minerals and trace elements – some minerals help to strengthen and harden bone, and make it less susceptible to wear and tear. A good combination of minerals and trace elements is boron, zinc, copper, magnesium, manganese, and molybdenum. Supplements containing these ingredients are available for pets.

OTHERS

Copper is a natural anti-arthritic remedy, so placing a copper collar or chain on your pet is a useful and simple way of guarding against, or treating, arthritis.

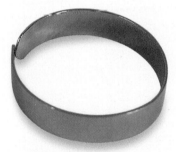

A copper collar can be used as a guard against arthritis as well as a treatment.

Arthritic pets may be unwilling to move and prefer to lie down, however do encourage exercise.

Sprains and strains

CAUSES

• injury or accident

SIGNS AND SYMPTOMS

• lameness
• joint or muscle pain and swelling

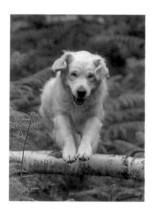

Active, playful animals are more prone to stumble and damage a ligament or tendon.

DOS AND DON'TS

Do rest the patient until the symptoms have gone, unless instructed to give exercise by your veterinarian.

Do remember that acupuncture and the other therapies highlighted on page108 may be appropriate.

Treatment of sprains requires drugs to reduce the swelling and, most importantly, rest.

The heading "Sprains and strains" covers a whole range of minor injuries, including pulled muscles, inflamed tendons, and stretched ligaments.

The symptoms vary according to the condition, but you should look out for lameness, sudden onset of pain, dislike of being touched or stroked in a particular area, and swelling.

Sprains and strains can be caused by accidents. They are obviously more likely to occur in energetic, hyperactive animals than those that are inactive. However, even the least active pet can stumble and damage a ligament or tendon.

Any major accidents or injuries obviously need rapid veterinary attention, as does lameness that is still present after 24 hours. Some ligament damage can be serious – the cruciate ligament, a ligament in the knee joint, will sometimes rupture completely. This may need surgery or long-term treatment to resolve.

Although in theory support bandages and dressings are useful for sprains and strains, in practice it is very difficult to keep such dressings on pets, especially smaller pets. Never put pressure dressings on limbs yourself – bandaging pets in these situations is best left to experts!

REMEDIES

Treatment in the short term comprises rest and restriction of movement. Apply an ice pack as soon as possible to reduce swelling, pain, and inflammation. After the first three days, warm applications in the form of an infra-red lamp or warm water bathing will help to speed healing.

PHYSIOTHERAPY
Physiotherapy will be useful (see page 58) if lameness persists longer than a week.

AROMATHERAPY
Massage of diluted essential oils will relieve pain and discomfort and help return normal function. **Aniseed**, **West Indian bay, camphor, clove bud, black pepper,** and **marjoram** are all beneficial for sprains and strains.

HERBAL
Witch hazel – applied directly to the sprained area will soothe and heal.
Comfrey – aids healing.

CRYSTAL AND GEM ESSENCES
Zircon helps stimulate repair of damaged ligaments, muscles, and tendons, especially cartilage injuries.

HOMEOPATHY
Arnica – should always be given immediately after a sprain or strain occurs. It will minimize bruising and swelling, and help the damaged tissue return to normal use more rapidly.
Hypericum – if there is severe pain at the site of the injury, Hypericum is a natural painkiller.
Ruta grav. – this is a specific homeopathic remedy for sprains and can be given after an initial course of Arnica to complete the healing process.
Bellis per. – if there is deep muscular bruising as part of the injury.
Rhus tox. – for persistent sprains that are taking a long time to heal; give Rhus tox and Ruta grav. together.

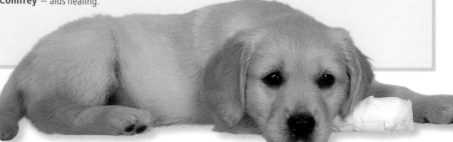

Myositis

Myositis is an inflammation of muscle tissue. Its symptoms are pain and swelling in one or more muscles, and discomfort in using muscles. In severe cases, there is distinct unwillingness or inability to use muscles.

It is caused by: bacterial infections – usually through untreated wounds; parasites – toxoplasma and neospora are two parasites that can damage and inflame muscle tissue in dogs and cats; immune disease – in some immune or auto-immune conditions, muscles will become painful and swollen.

• Myositis is mainly a disease of dogs and cats.

• Hamsters are affected by a problem called cage paralysis. They are completely or partially paralysed by this condition. It can be caused by injury, from simple lack of exercise, or by a myositis-type syndrome that is a result of vitamin D and E deficiency. Supplementation of the diet with these vitamins will cure the condition if this is the cause.

A particular form of myositis (eosinophilic myositis) affects the muscles of the jaw. This causes intense pain and difficulty in opening the mouth and the affected pet, usually a dog, may run a temperature. Following an acute bout of eosinophilic myositis, the muscles may atrophy, leading to long-term problems in opening the mouth and using the jaws. The cause of this condition is not certain, but may be an allergic reaction to an unknown allergen, or a viral infection.

Atrophic myositis – the gradual wasting of the jaw muscles – can occur as a result of eosinophilic myositis, or independently of it.

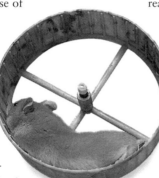

Lack of exercise can lead to cage paralysis. Always provide some means of exercise.

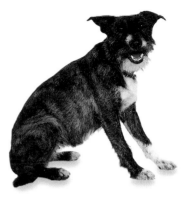

Myositis most commonly occurs in cats and dogs.

CAUSES

- bacterial infection
- parasites
- bacterial infection

SIGNS AND SYMPTOMS

- pain and swelling in muscles
- discomfort using muscles
- unwillingness/inability to use muscles

Gently massage basil into the affected area.

REMEDIES

Underlying causes such as injury, infection, or parasites should be treated. Conventional treatment would be steroids in most cases, but natural medicines may reduce or remove the need for these drugs, which are likely to cause side-effects if used long term.

AROMATHERAPY
Massaging diluted essential oils over damaged areas of muscle will be soothing and healing. Since the area may be painful, be very gentle, and do not continue massage if it is too uncomfortable for the patient.
Aniseed, basil, camomile (Roman or German), **ginger, lemongrass, marjoram, nutmeg, pepper, pine,** and **thyme** all have a healing action in cases of myositis.

HERBAL
White willow bark – this natural aspirin will minimize the pain of myositis.
Feverfew – will relieve the pain and also help if the patient is running a temperature.

CRYSTAL AND GEM ESSENCES
Rutilated quartz – will relieve the pain of myositis.
Zircon – will encourage healing of damaged muscle.

HOMEOPATHY
Bellis per. – ideal for deep muscular bruising and inflammation.
Arnica – for the tissue damage caused by myositis.

Aconite – for the inflammation, if given at the first signs of myositis.
Causticum – for long-term stiffness in muscles following myositis.
Silicea – for any scarring in muscles after an acute bout of myositis.
Mag. phos. – for muscle cramp pains.

OTHERS
Physiotherapy and **acupuncture** are two beneficial therapies to make use of, where available.
Ice packs at the time of acute myositis will minimize tissue damage.

Hip dysplasia (HD)

This is a developmental defect of the hip joints, affecting large breeds of dogs, particularly German shepherd dogs, labradors, and retrievers. One or both hips become progressively malformed, leading eventually to arthritis.

The symptoms vary from a mild rolling gait when walking to severe stiffness and lameness of the hindquarters, causing difficulty with mobility. Symptoms may occur at a few months of age, or not until the dog is fully grown and mature.

It is caused by a genetic abnormality, but the degree of severity is affected by environmental factors. Poor or imbalanced nutrition, and over-exercise as a growing puppy, can exacerbate symptoms.

REMEDIES

Severe cases may need to be treated by surgery, but normally anti-inflammatory and painkilling remedies are sufficient.
Natural medicines are effective treatments for hip dysplasia, and if given from a young age can stop symptoms from worsening.

HOMEOPATHY
Colocynth – specific for the symptoms of HD.
Calc. carb. – for the heavily built dog with hip dysplasia.
Calc. phos. – for lighter-boned, thinner dogs with hip dysplasia.

HERBAL
White willow will relieve the discomfort of hip dysplasia.

NUTRITIONAL
Vitamins C, B-complex, and **E** are all useful supplements.

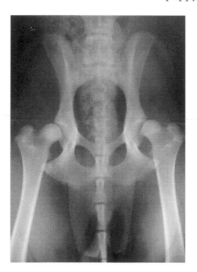

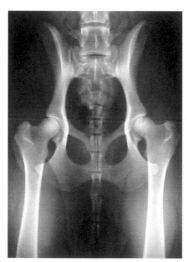

This dog has hip dysplasia. The joints are malformed and arthritis is developing.

This x-ray shows the hips of a healthy dog. The joints are perfectly normal.

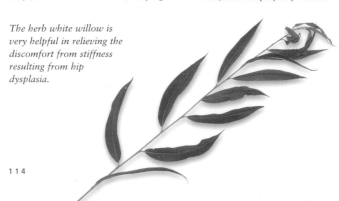

The herb white willow is very helpful in relieving the discomfort from stiffness resulting from hip dysplasia.

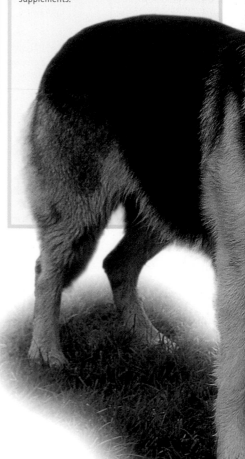

Dislocation

A dislocation, also known as subluxation, occurs when a bone comes out of its socket or other attachment to the next bone.

The symptoms are sudden and obvious lameness, or the inability to use one leg. The dislocated joint will usually be visibly misshapen, although this may not be so obvious in the case of hip joints.

It is usually caused by injuries, but in rare cases may be congenital – certain joints are malformed from birth, or develop so in adolescence, and consequently dislocate easily. This is particularly the case in the knee caps of small breeds of dogs, such as miniature poodles and Yorkshire terriers. Joints already affected by hip dysplasia, a condition causing malformation of hip joints in large breeds such as German shepherds, are more likely to dislocate.

Miniature breeds are prone to dislocation of the knee caps.

CAUSES

- injury
- congenital abnormality

SIGNS AND SYMPTOMS

- sudden, obvious lameness
- inability to use one leg
- visibly misshapen joint

Hip dysplasia usually affects large breeds of dog such as German shepherds, labradors, and retrievers.

REMEDIES

As far as treatment is concerned, physical replacement of the dislocated bone will need to be performed by your veterinarian. Natural remedies will help to prevent recurrence (dislocated joints often redislocate easily because supporting ligaments and other tissues have been stretched and weakened) and will minimize pain and bruising at the site.

HERBAL
Apply **witch hazel** lotion over the dislocation to soothe, cool and speed healing.

CRYSTAL AND GEM ESSENCES
Sapphire will help ease the pain following dislocations.
Zircon will help heal and repair damaged tissues after dislocations.

HOMEOPATHY
Arnica is ideal to give at the time of dislocation injuries to minimize bruising and swelling.
Aconite is good to minimize the shock that can accompany dislocation.
Rhus tox. and **Ruta grav.** given together will help speed healing.

OTHERS
Ice packs at the time of injury will minimize swelling and make the process of returning the bone to its socket much easier.

Following dislocation of a joint, sapphire can be used to ease the pain.

Other bone conditions

• dietary imbalance

• bones are soft and deformed

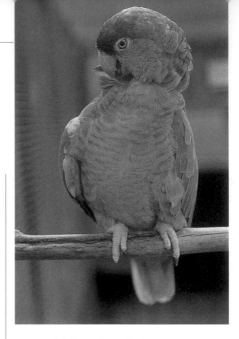

A mineral deficient diet in birds will cause the soft bone condition osteomalacia.

There is a group of bone conditions, all related to incorrect development or nourishment of growing bone. In the majority of the following conditions, therapies such as acupuncture, osteopathy, chiropractic physiotherapy, and magnetic therapy will be appropriate. Other specific natural medicines are shown separately. Always check the animal's diet and get veterinary advice on any necessary changes.

FERRET OSTEODYSTROPHY

This is a calcium deficiency caused by an imbalanced all-meat diet in ferrets. It occurs when the ferret is 6–12 weeks old and affects the entire litter. The ferrets become unable to stand because their bones have become soft and deformed.

OSTEOMALACIA

This condition is a failure of developing bone tissue to absorb sufficient minerals to harden the bone. It appears most often in birds and dogs. The affected birds have bent legs, with swollen joints, and cannot grip perches properly. Affected dogs are lame, have visibly deformed bones, and bones fracture easily. The most usual cause is an imbalanced diet – too much vitamin D, or too little calcium.

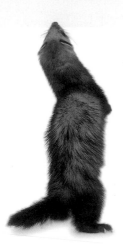

An imbalanced, calcium deficient diet will cause a soft bone condition in young ferrets – known as ferret osteodystrophy.

• dietary imbalance

• in birds: bent legs, swollen joints
• in dogs: lameness, deformed bones; bones fracture easily

REMEDIES

FERRET OSTEODYSTROPHY

Dietary adjustment, if introduced early enough, will normally resolve symptoms.

HOMEOPATHY
Calc. phos. – helps the body absorb minerals efficiently.
Calc. fluor. – strengthens bones.

NUTRITIONAL
Boron in supplements is especially effective.

OSTEOMALACIA

Treat urgently with vitamin and mineral supplements, especially **calcium.**

HOMEOPATHY
Calc. phos. – helps the body absorb minerals efficiently.
Calc. fluor. – strengthens bones.

OSTEOCHONDROSIS

ACUPUNCTURE
This is particularly beneficial for osteochondrosis.

HOMEOPATHY
Calc. carb. – for big-boned, heavy dogs.
Calc. phos. – for thinner, lighter dogs.
Calc. fluor. – to strengthen bones.

HERBAL
Feverfew – for pain in joints.
Greenleaf herbs (nettles, dandelion, parsley) – to remove toxins from joints.

Lavender is soothing.

OSTEOCHONDROSIS

This illness is a disturbance of the hardening of the growth plates (the growing ends of the bones in the joints). Small flakes of cartilage may detach from the bone, causing discomfort and lameness. Osteochondrosis usually occurs in the shoulder, elbow, or hock (ankle) joints.

Larger breeds of dogs are affected – their joints are stiff and uncomfortable when moved, and they are often thickened. The cause of osteochoncrosis may be too rapid growth in heavy breeds, or dietary imbalance.

NUTRITIONAL OSTEODYSTROPHY

This condition occurs in young, growing tortoises, terrapins, and reptiles. Nutritional osteodystrophy is often found in terrapins fed an all-meat or fish fillet diet. Tortoises

Nutritional osteodystrophy will cause spinal degeneration in reptiles.

suffering from this condition have a domed or pyramid appearance to the shell, their beak is deformed, and their back legs splay out backward. Reptiles, mainly lizards, develop swollen legs and weakness or paralysis due to spinal degeneration.

METAPHYSEAL OSTEOPATHY

This is seen at 3–6 months of age in dogs, almost always "giant" breeds. Symptoms include enlarged and painful joints, high temperature, and bleeding from gums. Its cause is usually too much calcium.

NUTRITIONAL OSTEODYSTROPHY

CAUSES

- developmental defect
- poor diet and overexercise can exacerbate symptoms

SIGNS AND SYMPTOMS

- from mild rolling gait to severe stiffness and lameness of hindquarters

METAPHYSEAL OSTEODYSTROPHY

CAUSES

- excessive calcium intake

SIGNS AND SYMPTOMS

- enlarged, painful joints
- high temperature
- bleeding from gums

An excess of calcium can cause a temperature and swollen joints in immature "giant" breeds.

AROMATHERAPY
Lavender to soothe pain and inflammation.

NUTRITIONAL
Glucosamines to help build healthy cartilage in joints.

NUTRITIONAL OSTEODYSTROPHY

HOMEOPATHY
Calc. phos. – improves absorption of minerals.
Calc. fluor. – strengthens bones.

NUTRITIONAL
Terrapins – avoid red meat; give whole fish as well as mineral and vitamin supplements.
Tortoises – add vitamin and mineral supplements to all meals by sprinkling them on fruit and vegetables.
Reptiles – calcium supplementation required.

METAPHYSEAL OSTEODYSTROPHY

NUTRITIONAL
Vitamin C will help damaged joints and gums.

HOMEOPATHY
Phosphorus – a remedy for bone destruction and bleeding gums.
Calc. phos. – improves correct mineral absorption.

HERBAL
Feverfew – relieves pain in joints.
Lavender essential oil – soothes and relieves inflammation.

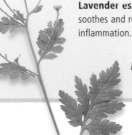

Feverfew

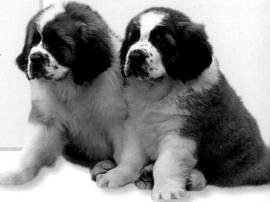

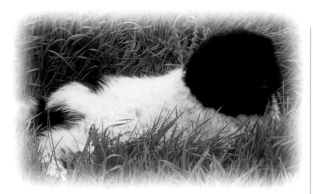

Young, growing dogs can be affected by panosteitis, which causes a thickening of the limb bones.

PANOSTEITIS

This condition is a localized thickening of limb bones in young, growing dogs, mainly the larger breeds.

The symptoms are recurring lameness and shifting from leg to leg. This maybe accompanied by a high temperature.

The cause is unknown but may be dietary. Avoid oversupplementing with minerals and vitamin D.

OSTEOMYELITIS

This is a bacterial infection in the bone tissue. The symptoms that manifest are local swelling, pain, and a high temperature. As the infection develops, pus may be evident. This will be oozing through the skin from the bone below.

Osteomyelitis is most commonly the result of an infected injury (for example, from another animal) or from the bacteria spreading to the bones via the bloodstream.

SPONDYLOSIS

This is a form of spinal arthritis, in which extra bone becomes laid down around the spinal vertebrae, gradually fusing them together. It is a problem mainly of large breeds of dogs.

The symptoms are a stiff, painful spine and weakness or paralysis of one or more limbs. Affected patients have difficulty in getting up.

Aging is the main cause. Occasionally it occurs after an infection, and in cats it can be caused by an excessive intake of vitamin A.

An x-ray will be required to confirm a diagnosis of spondylosis. This is the case with the majority of bone and joint conditions.

PANOSTEITIS

CAUSES

- dietary imbalance

SIGNS AND SYMPTOMS

- recurring lameness, shifting from leg to leg
- high temperature

OSTEOMYELITIS

CAUSES

- bacterial infection
- injury

SIGNS AND SYMPTOMS

- local swelling
- pain
- high temperature
- pus may be visible

REMEDIES

PANOSTEITIS

ACUPUNCTURE
This is especially helpful for pain control.

HERBAL
Feverfew – for pain in bones.

HOMEOPATHY
Belladonna – for high temperature and pain.

NUTRITIONAL
Vitamin C – helps normal bone development.

OSTEOMYELITIS

Treat with antibiotic therapy or the following:

HOMEOPATHY
Arnica – at the time of injury, Arnica will speed healing and minimize the likelihood of infection.

Hepar. sulph. – the classic homeopathic anti-infection remedy.
Silicea – to help drive infection and diseased fragments of bone out of the body.

HERBAL
Feverfew – for pain and inflammation.
Comfrey – to help heal damaged bone.

SPONDYLOSIS

All the treatments for arthritis (pages 110–111) will be beneficial as well as the following:

ACUPUNCTURE
Especially useful, this will provide pain relief.

HOMEOPATHY
Hypericum – for the pain and discomfort.
Causticum – for the "tearing, drawing" pains and the stiffness.

DISC PROTUSION

Otherwise known as a slipped disc, this is a degeneration of the shock-absorbing intervertebral disc, a pad of thick tissue between each bone of the spine. When the disc weakens and degenerates, it can move and begin to protrude from its position between the bones of the spine and consequently press on the spinal cord.

The symptoms are pain (which may be acute and agonising) and variable degrees of weakness or paralysis of one or more limbs. There may be a loss of bladder or bowel control in severe cases.

Disc protusion may follow an injury or may be a spontaneous protrusion as the disc "wears out." It is almost solely a problem of dogs, but is occasionally seen in ferrets. Particularly likely to be affected are long-backed dogs such as dachshunds, Pekingese, and middle-aged and older animals. The neck and mid or lower back are more commonly affected.

Disc protusion in its severest form is an absolute emergency and surgery may be

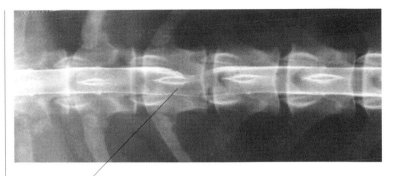

X-ray showing the protusion of the shock-absorbing intervertebral disc.

necessary to prevent permanent paralysis. Any symptoms of severe neck or back pain or of sudden onset paralysis in one or more legs must be seen as soon as possible by your veterinarian. In these cases give natural medicines for collapse and shock (see page 182) while awaiting veterinary attention. Following initial emergency treatment for disc protusion, or in less acute cases where simple conventional anti-inflammatory or painkillers are being prescribed, natural medicines can minimize pain and discomfort, and promote healing and strengthening.

DISC PROTUSION

CAUSES

- injury
- spontaneous protrusion as disc "wears out"

SIGNS AND SYMPTOMS

- pain
- weakness or paralysis of one or more limbs
- possible loss of bladder or bowel control

REMEDIES

ACUPUNCTURE
This relaxes muscles, relieves pain, and promotes healing at the site of damage.

AROMATHERAPY
Lavender, rosemary, eucalyptus, thyme, and **marjoram** will relieve pain, stiffness and tension. Do not massage over the damaged area, as this may be too painful. Use by diffusion, or massage well away from the painful spot.

HERBAL
White willow and **feverfew** will help with pain relief.
Greenleaf herbs will speed healing by removing toxins from the area.
Skullcap and **valerian** will calm the anxiety and stress which many dogs experience.

FLOWER AND GEM REMEDIES
Grapefruit – promotes healing of spinal damage of all kinds.

HOMEOPATHY
Hypericum – for pain relief.
Arnica – at the time of protrusion, this minimizes bruising and trauma.
Nux vomica – relieves the muscular pain and tension.

CRYSTALS AND GEM ESSENCES
Sapphire and **zircon** promote healing of damaged spinal tissues.

Dachshunds and other long-backed dogs are prone to disc protusion.

DOS AND DON'TS

If a severe disc protusion is suspected, do keep your pet as immobile as possible until seen by your veterinarian. Movement could damage the spinal cord more.

Don't forget that disc problems often recur. Get advice about long-term treatment, such as acupuncture, which can help prevent it recurring.

Chronic Degenerative Radiculomyelopathy

CAUSES

- degeneration of nerves supplying hindquarters

SIGNS AND SYMPTOMS

- loss of strength in hind legs
- swaying and weakness
- eventual inability to stand
- incontinence in later stages

Chronic Degenerative Radiculomyelopathy (CDRM) is a disease affecting the spinal cord of large breeds of dogs, mainly German shepherds. The main nerves supplying the hindquarters slowly degenerate, resulting in gradual paralysis and loss of sensation. Primarily a nerve disease, its symptoms are musculoskeletal.

The symptoms are a loss of strength in the hind legs, swaying and weakness when walking, "knuckling" (a turning-under of the feet), and an eventual inability to stand. The hind leg muscles begin to waste and there may be bladder or bowel incontinence in the later stages.

With CDRM, the body attacks its own tissues – in this case, the outer protective sheath of the nerve fibers. Many dogs affected by CDRM may also be suffering from arthritis, and from hip dysplasia. Once diagnosed, these conditions may need treatment in addition to CDRM.

REMEDIES

CDRM is a progressive condition and is not curable; there is no specific conventional treatment. Natural medicines are often effective in slowing down the rate of progression, and sometimes in stabilizing the condition for a period.

AROMATHERAPY
Juniper and **lavender** help relieve symptoms.

PHYSIOTHERAPY
Should always be used if available – it helps keep muscles working and slows down progression of the disease.

ACUPUNCTURE
Slows down weakening and onset of paralysis of muscles.

HOMOEOPATHY
Conium – specifically for the symptoms of paralysis, occurring from the hind end forwards.
Plumbum – helps any condition where nerve damage is present.

HERBAL
Ginkgo – improves circulation to weakened tissues.
Grapeseed extract – promotes healing in all chronic diseases of this nature.
Ginseng – improves stamina and ability of weakened muscles to function.

NUTRITIONAL
Oils – **blackcurrant seed oil**, **borage oil**, and **evening primrose oil** all contain fatty acids found in the degenerating nerve sheath. These oils help to slow down deterioration.
Vitamin E – give 2000 iu daily for affected patients. High dose vitamin E reduces the inflammation where the nerves are deteriorating and slows the progression of CDRM.
Vitamin C – works well in combination with vitamin E, acting as an antioxidant to reduce damage to nerve tissue.
Vitamin B-Complex – B vitamins help in nerve regeneration. High potency B-complex should be given (up to 100 mg daily of most B vitamins).
Selenium – in combination with vitamins E and C. Selenium is a potent antioxidant, therefore reducing damage to nerve tissue at the site of degeneration.
Coenzyme Q10 – helps minimize muscle wastage.
Two other nutritional supplements – **acetyl cysteine** and **aminocaproic acid** – have been reported as being beneficial in cases of CDRM. These are antioxidant, neuroprotective agents. At the time of writing, there is not sufficient information available on their true effectiveness.

PHYSIOTHERAPY
Together with exercise, this is vital. The muscles must be kept moving as much as possible to slow down wastage.
Swimming is ideal.

Physiotherapy helps to slow down the progression of CDRM and maintain muscular function.

Cancer

Cancer can develop in any tissue of the body. Some cancers – such as skin tumors – are visible and obvious, others may go unnoticed until they are quite large. The incidence of cancer in pets seems to be increasing – partly because many pets are living longer, but also because of immune system damage. Many cases of cancer occur in quite young pets, so age is not necessarily a major factor.

Natural therapies can be effective in controlling cancer, sometimes in obtaining remission, and always ensuring a pet affected by cancer feels better and suffers fewer symptoms. In a terminal case, they can ease the pet through the last few days or weeks, and make a natural, pain-free death more likely. Natural medicines can be given alongside conventional treatments – they can help prevent recurrence of cancer after surgery, help reduce the side-effects of chemotherapy while not interfering with the beneficial effects, and often their use means lower doses of conventional drugs can be administered. They are also compatible with any conventional drugs. However, some chemotherapy agents, especially steroids, will reduce the effectiveness of some natural medicines (particularly the effect of homeopathic remedies).

CAUSES

- weakness in immune system

SIGNS AND SYMPTOMS

These vary with the type of cancer, look for:
- lumps and growths – new, unusual, or fast-growing
- weakness and anemia
- loss of appetite
- loss of energy

REMEDIES

Since many cancers occur because of a weakness in the immune system, which allows the cancer cells to multiply, all the remedies to boost the immune system mentioned in the previous section will be useful in treating cancer.

AROMATHERAPY
Rosemary and **ylang ylang** are revitalizing and act as a tonic and a boost to the body's natural powers to attack cancer.
Bergamot and **sandalwood** help to counter the debility and weakness of terminal cancer.
Fennel – use if there is nausea and vomiting following chemotherapy.

HERBAL
Yellow dock, **garlic**, **nettles**, **myrrh**, **cleavers**, **thyme**, **poke root**, and **plantain** have all been shown to have anticancer activity. **Garlic** is especially useful in that it also reduces the risk of secondary infections. **Mistletoe extract**, injected directly into the tumor

Cancer can also affect very young animals.

has given good results in many cases, often shrinking the tumor considerably.
Red clover and **autumn crocus** have also been effective in controlling tumors.

ACUPUNCTURE
Some acupuncture points are stimulating to the body's mechanisms of attacking cancerous cells.

FLOWER AND GEM REMEDIES
Crab apple is a good cleansing and detoxifying remedy, and is especially useful when chemotherapy is being administered.
Hornbeam strengthens weakened animals.
Olive will help pets that seem to be giving in to the condition.

HOMEOPATHY
Hydrastis – for the early stages of most cancers, increasing the likelihood of remission. It will also help to reduce pain.
Arsen. alb. – helps relieve pain and suffering in terminal stages of cancer.
Viscum alb. – useful for reducing growth rate.
Carcinosin – for tumors in mammary glands and the skin.
Conium – for tumors in the older pet. The constitutional remedy for all cancers.

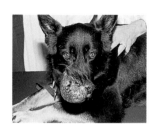

Cancerous skin tumors can develop into large growths.

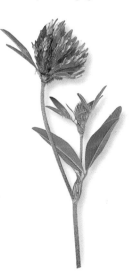

Red clover has been found effective in controlling cancer tumors.

Epilepsy and convulsions

CAUSES

- epilepsy: often hereditary
- convulsions: epilepsy, poisoning, infection, eclampsia, kidney failure, injury

SIGNS AND SYMPTOMS

- sudden loss of consciousness
- violent muscle spasms
- "paddling" or rigid legs
- frothing mouth
- loss of bladder or bowel control

Epilepsy is a specific disease of the brain causing intermittent, but repeated convulsions. It is an abnormal electrical discharge in the brain and is often hereditary; it is also a permanent condition. Convulsions are a set of symptoms that can be caused by epilepsy, but also by other factors. All epileptic pets have convulsions; but not all convulsions are necessarily caused by epilepsy.

Convulsions (also known as fits, or seizures) are very frightening to see. The affected pet loses consciousness suddenly – often without any warning. Some or all muscles go into violent spasms, legs may be held out rigidly, or go into a repeated paddling movement. The affected pet may froth at the mouth, and may lose control of bowel or bladder during the fit. A convulsion may last a few seconds, or several minutes. Convulsions caused by epilepsy are often followed by a period of confusion, lack of coordination, loss of sight, restlessness, and a strong desire to eat or drink.

Epileptic pets sometimes have minor episodes called "petit mals" – as opposed to a full fit, which is known as a "grand mal." In a petit mal the pet may not lose consciousness, but simply stops what he or she is doing, looks "blank" for a few seconds, and then suddenly "comes to" and carries on. The majority of epileptic fits occur while, or just after, the pet is asleep or resting. Some pets will show signs they are about to have a fit – look a little confused, or become restless or anxious.

The causes of epilepsy are unknown, although it is often hereditary.

Convulsions can have various causes:
- Poisoning.
- Infections – fits can be the symptom of various infections.
- Eclampsia – in bitches feeding young puppies.
- Kidney failure – in severe kidney disease, fits may occur.
- Injury – especially head injuries.
- Although reptiles rarely suffer convulsions, water snakes fed on frozen fish, or snakes fed on frozen chicks may develop thiamine (B vitamin) deficiency which can lead to seizures. Dietary change is usually all that is required.
- Most convulsions occur in dogs and cats, with dogs being particularly prone. The incidence of epilepsy in dogs is probably as high as that in humans.

Fits are usually intermittent, but sometimes a pet will go into a continuous series of fits. This is known as "status epilepticus" and is life-threatening. Immediate veterinary attention is required.

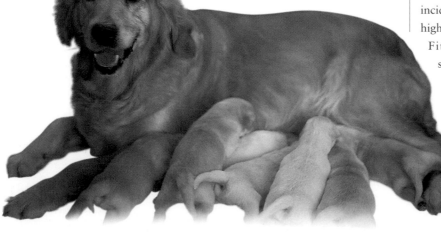

Convulsions will sometimes occur in bitches that are feeding puppies. This is usually due to the post-whelping condition of eclampsia.

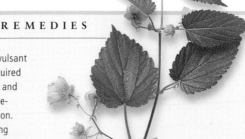

Hops will soothe and calm the nervous system.

REMEDIES

Conventional treatment prescribes anticonvulsant drugs. Often, higher doses of drugs are required to control the convulsions as time goes by, and the drugs are likely to have undesirable side-effects, liver damage being the most common. In non-epileptic causes of fits, the underlying problems must be diagnosed and treated. Natural medicines can minimize the side-effects of conventional drugs, and also treat the fits themselves. With natural medicines, the dose rate of conventional anticonvulsants can often be reduced, or even eliminated.

AROMATHERAPY
Lavender, camomile, melissa, ylang ylang, rose, and **neroli** will all help reduce fitting.

FLOWER AND GEM REMEDIES
Diamond, Chicago peace rose, and **nasturtium** will all help to prolong the periods between fits.

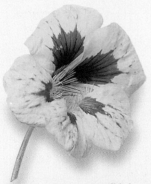

Nasturtium will help to reduce the frequency of fits.

HERBAL
Skullcap and **valerian** – this combination is ideal for epilepsy, especially in pets that have a tendency to be anxious or nervous.
Hops – another soothing, calming remedy for the nervous system.

CRYSTAL AND GEM ESSENCES
Brown agate and **jet** both help minimize intensity of fits.

HOMEOPATHY
Belladonna – helps soothe pets after a fit, especially if pupils remain dilated.
Cicuta virosa – if the head tends to be stretched back or to the side during a fit.
Stramonium – if the pet falls to the left side repeatedly.
Ignatia – if fits seem to be brought on by stress or emotional upset.
Aconite – if fits are brought on by shock or fear.
Bufo – if fits always seem to start during sleep or while the animal is resting.
Camomile – if fits are brought on by teething pains in young animals.
Phosphorus – if fits start after sudden bangs or noises and if head-twitching occurs between fits.
Scutellaria – for hyperactive pets with strange behavior patterns.
Zinc – for pets sensitive to noise; head falls to the left during a fit.

COLOR THERAPY
Blue is a calming color for pets suffering convulsions.

Water snakes may have seizures as a result of Vitamin B deficiency.

DOS AND DON'TS

Do keep pets quiet and in a darkened room during a fit.

Don't try to put anything in the mouth – the tongue rarely gets bitten, but you might be.

Do watch for situations or emotions that trigger fits and try to avoid them.

Don't ring your vet every time a fit occurs. If epilepsy has been diagnosed, the only emergency situation is if status epilepticus occurs.

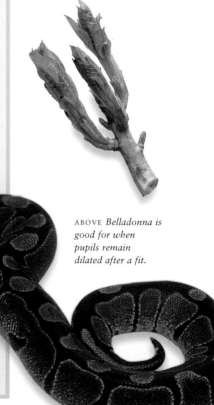

ABOVE *Belladonna is good for when pupils remain dilated after a fit.*

Meningitis and encephalitis

Meningitis is an inflammation of the tissues around the brain. Encephalitis is an inflammation of the brain tissue itself.

The symptoms and causes are similar for both. Symptoms are a stiff neck, pressing head against something hard and solid, unwilling to have head touched or stroked, high temperature, unusual behavior (aggression, depression, excitability), swaying, falling, convulsions, and hindquarter paralysis.

Both can be caused by infections (canine distemper, rabies, bacteria). Parasites can also be a cause. Brain tumors can bring about symptoms of encephalitis. Dogs that were affected by, but recovered from, distemper in their youth sometimes show symptoms (known as "old dog encephalitis") in old age.

REMEDIES

Any condition of the brain needs rapid veterinary attention. Apart from any necessary conventional treatment required, and when any underlying causes such as infections have been treated, the following natural medicines will be most beneficial.

AROMATHERAPY
Lavender, camomile, rosemary, clary sage, and **marjoram** will all relieve symptoms.

HERBAL
Skullcap and **valerian**. This combination will relieve pain, distress, and discomfort.

FLOWER AND GEM REMEDIES
Rock rose will help when symptoms are acute. **Sapphire, nasturtium,** and **comfrey** are good in more chronic cases.

Comfrey

Neuritis

Neuritis is an inflammation of a nerve, or a group of nerves. The symptoms are persistent localized pain, irritation, or itchiness, resulting in frequent licking, scratching, or biting at the affected area. It can be caused by:

- Injuries – superficial nerves are often damaged in severe wounds and lacerations.
- Nerve tumor – dogs and cats, but rarely.
- Pressure – for example a trapped nerve as in spondylosis (see page 118).
- Excessive facial itchiness in dogs may be nerve inflammation (trigeminal neuralgia).
- Excessive biting and licking at the site of an operation may be due to inflammation of a nerve injured during surgery.

REMEDIES

AROMATHERAPY
Lavender – massaged in or near the area.

FLOWER AND GEM REMEDIES
Star of Bethlehem – will calm distress.
Impatiens – for irritability or aggression.

HOMEOPATHY
Hypericum – for pain from damaged nerves.
Camomile – for the irritable, niggly patient.
Passiflora – a calming, soothing remedy.

PHYSIOTHERAPY
Ideal for neuritis, especially electrical stimulation therapy, laser treatment, and/or ultrasound.

Chorea

This is an involuntary twitching or shaking of muscles especially those in the jaw, legs, eyes, and ears. It may affect a single muscle, or a whole group of muscles. The commonest cause is as an aftereffect of distemper in dogs. Other causes include poisons and brain tumors. Some older dogs and cats seem to develop intermittent chorea as part of the natural aging process; one or more limbs may shake continuously.

CAUSES

- after effect of distemper
- poisoning
- brain tumors
- aging

SIGNS AND SYMPTOMS

- repeated twitching of muscles, especially in jaw, legs, eyes, and ears

---

REMEDIES

There is little in the way of conventional medicine to treat the symptoms of chorea. Any underlying cause should be treated.

AROMATHERAPY
Lavender, especially massaged (after dilution) at the site of the chorea.
Rosemary will also be helpful.
Both oils relax the muscles and so reduce twitching.

FLOWER AND GEM REMEDIES
Scleranthus is good for the lack of control that is symptomatic of chorea.

HERBAL
Skullcap with **valerian** act as a general calming, soothing herbal combination to reduce twitchiness and shaking.
Oats and **hops** will also help.
Ginkgo – improves circulation and blood supply.

Key Gaskell Syndrome

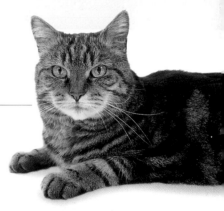

Cats can be affected by Key Gaskell syndrome, which affects the involuntary (autonomic) nerves.

This is a condition seen in cats. It affects only the involuntary nerves – such as the bowel muscles that move food along, or the muscles that dilate or constrict the pupils. In Key Gaskell syndrome, these muscles become weakened or paralysed.

The symptoms are dilated pupils, protrusion of a third eyelid across the eye, dry mouth, lack of appetite, difficulty in swallowing, vomiting, constipation, urine leakage or urine retention. Its cause is unknown, but is probably a viral infection.

CAUSES

- unknown

SIGNS AND SYMPTOMS

- dilated pupils
- protrusion of third eyelid
- dry mouth
- lack of appetite
- difficulty in swallowing
- vomiting
- constipation
- urine leakage or retention

REMEDIES

There is no direct conventional treatment. Supportive treatment comprises intravenous drips and general nursing care, which is vital in severe cases.

AROMATHERAPY
Basil and **marjoram** help lift a weak, depressed cat with Key Gaskell syndrome.

FLOWER AND GEM REMEDIES
Olive – for physical and mental exhaustion.

Gorse – for a cat that appears to be giving in to the condition.
Clematis – for the cat that seems to "go into a dream world."

HOMEOPATHY
Gelsemium – for nerve and muscle weakness.
Belladonna – for dry mouth and dilated pupils.
Opium – for weakness and constipation.
Calc. carb. – for big, heavy, overweight cats.

Vomiting

Vomiting is simply being sick – bringing the contents of the stomach up the wrong way.

Symptoms are rather self-evident! Vomiting may be intermittent, or in acute gastritis (inflammation of the stomach) can be persistent. Persistent vomiting is debilitating and the patient rapidly becomes weak and dehydrated. Some pets (dogs and cats) are sick quite easily, and the odd bout of vomiting is quite normal. Fish cannot vomit. Rabbits, rats, mice, guinea pigs, hamsters, and gerbils vomit very rarely, and it is a serious sign if they do seem to be vomiting. Any pet that is being sick frequently, needs rapid veterinary attention.

Vomiting can be caused by:

- Foreign bodies in the stomach, esophagus, or throat.
- Gastritis – inflammation of the stomach.
- Gastric ulcer – dogs are the most likely pets to be affected.
- Gastric dilatation/torsion – trying to vomit repeatedly, with little or nothing actually brought up.
- Tumor, polyps, or any type of growth in the stomach may cause vomiting.
- Drug reactions – some conventional drugs or certain antibiotics may cause stomach inflammation and vomiting.
- Irritants – swallowed accidentally, these can cause vomiting.
- Travel sickness.
- Infections – many bacterial and viral infections have vomiting as one of their symptoms.
- Internal disease – liver, kidney, and pancreatic disease often cause vomiting, as do diabetes mellitus and pyometra (an infection of the womb).

Travel sickness is often experienced in cars and will cause vomiting.

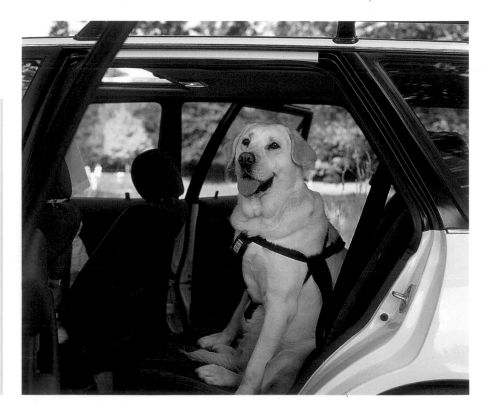

REMEDIES

Any specific known causes should be treated. Otherwise, conventional treatment consists of giving anti-emetic drugs (drugs that suppress the center in the brain controlling vomiting) and supportive treatment such as fluid replacement for the fluids lost in vomiting.

Natural remedies that can help include:

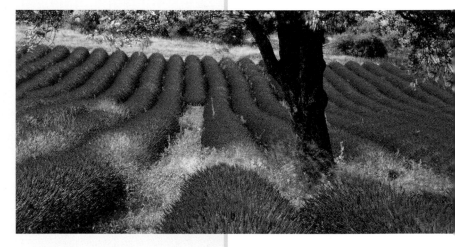

Lavender will relieve emotional upset.

AROMATHERAPY
Lavender – where vomiting is due to nervousness or emotional upset.
Peppermint – where vomiting is accompanied by high temperature or diarrhea, or is caused by travel sickness.
Ginger – very soothing and calming for the soreness of the stomach when repeated vomiting is going on.
Cardamon – where vomiting is caused by eating unsuitable foods.

Nutmeg kernal

Melissa – vomiting accompanied by colic in nervous animals.
Aniseed – vomiting with much wind and flatulence.
Nutmeg – vomiting with sluggish digestion, tendency to constipation.

HERBAL
Gentian root, St John's wort, and **peppermint** all soothe the stomach and relieve the inflammation which triggers vomiting.

HOMOEOPATHY
Apomorphine – this is a remedy made from a conventional drug, which is used to stimulate vomiting in pets that have swallowed toxins or poisons.
Apis mel. – mouth is dry, the vomiting is caused by an allergic reaction, the patient will feel better out in the open air.
Arsen. alb. – usually vomiting occurs in conjunction with diarrhea. A good food poisoning remedy. Patient is restless, wants to be warm, and wants to drink water little and often – not a lot at one time.

Phosphorus – vomiting very soon after eating food, may bring up blood.
Nux vomica – for vomiting that occurs soon after eating rich food or other inappropriate food. For dogs that raid the larder, or scavenge entirely unsuitable foods. Usually constipated at the same time. Nux vomica also helps where there is post-operative vomiting.
Ipecac. – simple regurgitation of food (often useful for birds that regurgitate food, although this may occur for behavioral reasons). Also suits intermittent vomiting of slimy material, and reduces retching and discomfort between bouts of vomiting.
Merc. sol. – yellow vomit, patient is very thirsty, but drinking water will make the pet keep on vomiting.
Merc. cor. – as Merc. sol but more violent vomiting, with mucoid material brought up.
Veratrum alb. – immediate regurgitation of food, with frothy yellow vomit at other times.
Pulsatilla – vomiting alternating with diarrhea. Vomiting several hours after eating fatty food.

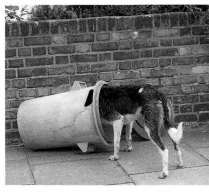

Scavenging in refuse containers and consuming unsuitable foods will often result in vomiting.

DOS AND DON'TS

Do treat vomiting with bloating of the abdomen as an emergency – it could be caused by gastric torsion.

Gentian root will soothe and relieve inflammation.

Foreign bodies

Swallowing non-food objects or foreign bodies, which become lodged in the stomach or intestines, is something that can happen to any pet, but is a more common occurence in some species.

The symptoms are vomiting, passing few or no feces, abdominal discomfort, depression, and dehydration.

There can be several causes – a variety of objects have been found in animals' digestive tracts. Among very many objects, dogs swallow bones (never feed cooked bones to dogs – they cannot digest them). Cats swallow needles, elastic bands, and fur balls – a collection of hair in the stomach swallowed while grooming. Rabbits also develop hair balls from excessive grooming.

Rabbits are prone to developing hair balls through excessive grooming or combing.

REMEDIES

With a firmly-lodged foreign body, surgery is often essential. Small foreign bodies, including hair balls, can be encouraged to move on their way through the digestive tract by giving a little liquid paraffin each day for a few days. Also use natural medicines.

HOMEOPATHY
Nux vomica – helps small foreign bodies on their way.
Ornithogallum tincture – good for foreign bodies in the stomach.
Colchicum – relaxes the spasm of intestinal muscles that may be preventing a foreign body from moving on.

HERBAL
Peppermint – a traditional and common remedy for soothing the digestive tract.

Intussusception

CAUSES

- excessive bowel muscle movement
- canine distemper
- tumors in intestine
- **in puppies:** worms

SIGNS AND SYMPTOMS

- vomiting
- diarrhea
- abdominal pain
- blood and mucus in feces

Intussusception can be the result of an overwhelming infestation of worms in immature animals.

This is where the intestine telescopes into itself due to excessive muscular contraction of the intestinal wall. This can follow severe diarrhea; be a consequence of distemper or intestinal tumors; and in puppies, it may occur when large numbers of worms are present. The intestine becomes obstructed and blood supply to the affected intestine is damaged.

Vomiting, diarrhea, abdominal pain, blood, and mucus in feces will occur.

REMEDIES

In severe cases, surgery is essential – the condition is life-threatening. If diagnosed or suspected at an early stage, the following natural medicines may be sufficient.

HOMEOPATHY
Colchicum and **colocynth** – to relieve excessive muscle spasm and movement.
Cina – if worms are the cause.
Nux vomica – as a digestive stabilizer.

HERBAL
Peppermint and **camomile** – to soothe and calm the digestive tract.

Peppermint calms and soothes the digestion.

Gastric torsion and dilation

In this condition, gas is formed in the stomach, causing a rapid swelling and increase in pressure. As the gas builds up and the stomach becomes more and more dilated, it may twist inside the abdomen, which then seals the gas inside – this is gastric torsion.

The symptoms are a visible, rapidly increasing swelling of the abdomen. Pain and discomfort arise, along with unsuccessful attempts to vomit.

The causes are not fully understood. It often occurs after a large meal has been taken, followed by exercise, and is mainly a problem of large breeds of dogs.

REMEDIES

In severe cases, this condition can be life-threatening and require surgery. Contact your veterinarian, but in the meantime use:

HOMEOPATHY
Ornithogallum tincture – good for all stomach pain and swelling.
Colocynth – relaxes muscles and helps prevent torsion (twisting).

HERBAL
Peppermint and **camomile** relieve inflammation in the digestive tract and help natural release of gas.

CAUSES

- these conditions are not fully understood – can occur after large meal followed by exercise

SIGNS AND SYMPTOM

- pain and discomfort
- unsuccessful attempts to vomit

Flatulence and colic

Flatulence is an excessive build-up of gas in the bowels, which is expelled in a fairly unmistakable way. Colic is the discomfort caused by the presence in the intestines of gas that has not been passed – although colic can also be caused by muscular spasms that occur when intussusception, foreign bodies, gastric dilation, or acute diarrhea are present.

The symptoms are abdominal pain, swelling of the abdomen, and the passage of gas from the anus. Both flatulence and colic are often caused by an imbalanced diet – too high- or too low-fiber diets are the commonest cause. Bowel infection, or any infection causing diarrhea, may also cause gas to form. Some breeds of dogs, especially Boxers, are prone to flatulence, and tortoises sometimes develop colic, which then causes the intestines to fill with gas.

REMEDIES

Treat underlying causes, then investigate to find the right diet. Add charcoal biscuits or granules to the diet – charcoal absorbs excess gas.

AROMATHERAPY
Angelica root, aniseed, cardamom, dill seed, fennel, marjoram, neroli, and **yarrow**

HERBAL
Camomile and **peppermint** – antiflatulent
Fennel – good for irritable bowels.

CRYSTAL AND GEM ESSENCES
Coral – helps settle upset bowels with excess gas production.

HOMEOPATHY
Carbo. veg. – an ideal remedy to minimize flatulence in dogs.
Lycopodium – suits thin pets that like sweet-tasting foods.

CAUSES

- dietary imbalance
- bowel infection

SIGNS AND SYMPTOMS

- **flatulence**: expulsion of bowel gas
- **colic**: discomfort caused by gas in intestines

Charcoal biscuits offer dietary relief of the symptoms of flatulence.

Liver disease

The liver is an essential part of the digestive process. It has many functions – producing enzymes needed for digestion, controlling the distribution of nutrients absorbed from the digestive tract, and detoxifying poisons. Liver disease may be acute and immediately life-threatening, as in hepatitis, or chronic and slowly developing, as in liver disease.

In acute liver disease, the symptoms are vomiting, abdominal pain, lack of appetite, high temperature, and possibly jaundice (yellowing of skin, eyes, and gums). In chronic liver disease, the symptoms may be minor at the start – eating less and fussily, less energy, weight loss. Later, jaundice may develop, there may be an increase in thirst, digestive upsets, vomiting or diarrhoea, sometimes ascites (excess fluid in the abdomen causing visible swelling).

Liver disease is caused by:
- Liver tumors.
- Infections – viruses can cause hepatitis.
- Poisons – any toxin absorbed by the body will rapidly reach the liver; if the liver is unable to neutralize it, liver damage results.
- Trauma – major accidents and injuries may damage the liver.
- Other diseases – including diabetes mellitus and Cushing's disease.
- Drugs – conventional drugs often cause liver damage; any long-term medication, especially anticonvulsants used for epilepsy.
- Cirrhosis – this is a scarring and shrinking of the liver, which can happen as a result of toxins or poisons (although rarely in animals, as it is a result of excessive alcohol intake in humans). Cirrhosis also occurs as a natural aging process in some pets.
- Congenital defects.
- A genetic defect in certain breeds of dogs – mainly Bedlington terriers – prevents affected animals' ability to reject copper from the body. Copper builds up in the liver, eventually causing liver damage.
- Immune system disease.

Liver disease is commonest in dogs and cats, but smaller pets can also be affected. The most frequent cause of liver disease in gerbils, hamsters, rats, and mice is Tyzzer's disease, a bacterial infection that causes acute diarrhea and liver damage.

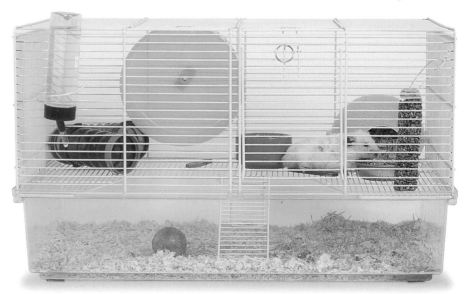

Tyzzer's disease is a frequent cause of diarrhea and liver damage in small animals.

REMEDIES

The liver is capable of regeneratin damaged tissue to a large extent. With the help of natural medicines, many pets are able to make a good recovery from liver disease. Treat any known underlying cause. Acute liver disease will need immediate veterinary attention. Diet is important – avoid fatty or rich foods and feed little and often rather than one large meal a day, so that the liver doesn't become overloaded. Get veterinary advice on the correct diet for the particular liver problem.

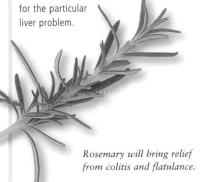

Rosemary will bring relief from colitis and flatulance.

AROMATHERAPY

Rosemary – for liver problems with jaundice. Patient prone to colitis and flatulence.

Carrot seed – liver disease with loss of appetite and abdominal pain.

Celery seed – jaundice with swollen liver.

Rose maroc – liver condition with nausea and vomiting. Good for lymphocytic cholangitis in cats.

Spanish sage – hepatitis with jaundice.

Yarrow – liver disease with constipation and abdominal pain.

FLOWER AND GEM REMEDIES

Crab apple – a detoxifying Bach Flower remedy for use following poisons or toxins.

Onyx – a liver support and clearing remedy, good for chronic liver disease.

HERBAL

Barberry – a liver tonic stimulates bile flow to improve digestion. Improves appetite and relieves constipation.

Burdock – for chronic liver disease, especially if accompanied by skin disease.

Dandelion – cleansing and detoxifying. Often used in combination with burdock for liver problems. Especially good for jaundice.

Elderberry – for liver and stomach disorders, especially if accompanied by circulatory problems.

Parsley piert – for liver disease, often with jaundice, and sometimes additional problems with stones or gravel in the bladder.

Yellow dock – for liver disorders associated with imbalanced diet, sluggish digestion, and constipation

Milk thistle – a superb liver support remedy. Helps treat all liver conditions, but is particularly useful to help protect the liver against damage from conventional medication, such as anticonvulsants in epileptic patients, or chemotherapeutic drugs in cancer patients.

CRYSTAL AND GEM ESSENCES

Amber – detoxifying, promotes liver function.

Yellow beryl – good for jaundice.

Coral – for liver and digestive disorders, especially where constipation and flatulence are a feature.

HOMEOPATHY

Aloe – useful where liver disease has occurred as a result of long-term dosing with conventional drugs. Improves circulation to liver and bowel. Diarrhea with mucus is often noticeable.

Berberis – jaundice and the passing of clay-coloured feces are prime indications for using berberis. There is a noticeable weakness and tenderness over the lower back and pelvic area. Often accompanied by kidney disease.

Chelidonium – lethargy and weakness; jaundice, vomiting, and yellow urine are present; whites of the eyes are particularly bright

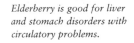

Elderberry is good for liver and stomach disorders with circulatory problems.

yellow. Feces yellow or clay-colored.

Iris vers. – for generally mild liver disease, loss of appetite, some abdominal discomfort, sometimes colicky pains. Often accompanied by pancreatic disease.

Lycopodium – liver inflammation with ascites (fluid in abdomen) and tendency to small, hard feces.

Nux vomica – sensitive and tender liver, constipation or hard stools, good for liver problems brought on by unsuitable foods, or poisons.

Phosphorus – acute liver disease with pain and vomiting.

NUTRITIONAL

Vitamins C and B-complex will help to promote liver function, and minimize damage.

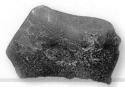

Amber will help with cleansing the liver and promotes normal liver function.

Pancreatic insufficiency

CAUSES

- follow-on from pancreatitis
- pancreatic degeneration

SIGNS AND SYMPTOMS

- diarrhea/flatulence
- coprophagia
- dry, harsh coat

Large breeds of dogs are more prone to pancreatic insufficiency.

The pancreas produces enzymes to help digest food traveling through the intestines and also produces insulin. Two conditions of the pancreas are found in pets – pancreatic insufficiency and pancreatitis.

In the case of pancreatic insufficiency, the pancreas is producing insufficient enzymes to digest food properly.

The symptoms are weight loss, increased appetite, diarrhea, coprophagia (eating feces), flatulence, and a dry harsh coat.

Pancreatic insufficiency tends to occur following pancreatitis or as a result of a degeneration of the pancreas, a feature of certain breeds of dogs, and one that seems to be congenital.

REMEDIES

Treat it in the following ways:

NUTRITIONAL
The missing enzymes can be added to the diet, but this must be on a permanent basis.

DIETARY
A low-fiber, moderate-fat diet, which must be highly digestible, is necessary. Consult your veterinarian as to the best balanced diet to give for any particular individual.

HOMEOPATHY
Iris vers. – helps promote normal pancreatic function.

FLOWER AND GEM REMEDIES
Topaz and **sugar beet** both help increase secretion of pancreatic enzymes.

CRYSTAL AND GEM ESSENCES
Sodalite stimulates glands, including the pancreas, to produce normal secretions.

Pancreatitis

CAUSES

- unknown – possibly excessive intake of fats
- sometimes follows surgery or long-term steroid use

SIGNS AND SYMPTOMS

- high temperature
- abdominal pain
- vomiting
- loss of appetite
- diarrhea

Pancreatitis is an inflammation of the pancreas and is a life-threatening condition. Fortunately, it is rarely seen by veterinarians, as it can be difficult to treat.

The symptoms are a high temperature, abdominal pain, vomiting, loss of appetite, and diarrhoea.

The causes are unknown, but may be to do with excessive intake of fats. Sometimes pancreatitis follows particularly high or long-term doses of steroids; or it may follow after surgery on the central nervous system. It is most common in overweight, middle-aged bitches.

REMEDIES

FLOWER AND GEM REMEDIES
Topaz and **sugar beet** help the pancreas return to normal function.

HOMOEOPATHY
Phosphorus – heals an inflamed pancreas.

NUTRITIONAL
Vitamins C and **B-complex** will enhance the healing process after pancreatitis.
Silicea – helps resolve scarring which may form after an acute bout of pancreatitis.
Iris vers. – stimulates normal pancreatic function after pancreatitis.

Constipation

Constipation is the infrequent passage of stools, or absence of defecation. The symptoms are: straining to pass feces or irregular (perhaps even absent) defecation. Stools that are passed are often hard and dry; sometimes they may be flattened or "ribbon-like."

It is caused by:

• Imbalanced diet – usually too little fiber or inappropriate foods.

• Growths – bowel tumors and polyps, which can cause obstructions in the bowel.

• Enlarged prostate – this will press upward on the rectum, producing thin, flattened, feces that are difficult to pass.

• Megacolon – a condition where the colon becomes enlarged, and unable to contract and push feces through it.

• Injuries – usually an indirect consequence of injuries to the pelvis, after major falls or the result of road traffic accidents. The pelvis, after healing, is narrowed, causing difficulty in feces passing through.

• Perineal hernia – a hernia on one or both sides of the anus, leading to weakness in the muscles of the area. Part of the rectum enters the herniated area, creating a "pocket" where feces collect.

• Rectal diverticulum – a condition where weakness in the wall of the rectum leads to the formation of "pouches" in which feces collect.

• Strictures – narrowings of the bowel caused by injuries or adhesions, which limit the amount of fecal material that can move through.

CAUSES

• dietary imbalance
• bowel tumors or polyps
• enlarged prostate
• megacolon
• injury
• rectal diverticulum
• strictures

SIGNS AND SYMPTOMS

• straining to pass feces
• irregular or absent defecation
• hard, dry stools

REMEDIES

Treat constipation with enemas in severe cases – these must be administered by your veterinary practice. Add fiber to the diet – bran is ideal. Young hamsters with constipation need extra green vegetables and fruit. Other suitable high-fiber products are dried fruit and psyllium husks. Liquid paraffin for very short periods is acceptable to help relieve constipation, but long-term use prevents the absorption of vitamins A, D, and E. Treat any underlying causes, such as prostate disease.

AROMATHERAPY
Fennel, marjoram, orange, and **yarrow** all help natural digestive function.

FLOWER AND GEM REMEDIES
Camphor relieves constipation.

CRYSTAL AND GEM ESSENCES
Coral improves bowel muscle tone.

HERBAL
Rhubarb and **cascara** are ideal mild laxatives.

Bearberry and **damiana** help restore tone to bowel muscles.

HOMEOPATHY
Sulfur – large, bulky stool, painful to pass, anus looks red and sore.
Silicea – stool comes part way out, then recedes again.
Calc. carb. – hard, chalky feces, especially after eating bones.
Nux vomica – constipation following operation.
Opium – lack of bowel movement.

ACUPUNCTURE
Can stimulate bowel muscles to function.

Rhubarb is ideal as a mild laxative to relieve the discomfort of constipation.

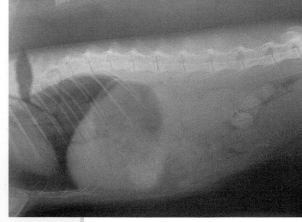

This pet is suffering from severe constipation – this can be seen as the large mass in the lower abdomen.

Diarrhea

CAUSES

- diet
- infection
- pancreatic insufficiency
- malabsorption syndrome
- colitis
- parasites
- poisons
- tumors

SIGNS AND SYMPTOMS

- abnormal consistency of feces
- passing of blood, mucus, or undigested food
- unpleasant smelling gas

Diarrhea is the single most common condition found in domestic pets.

Diarrhea is the single most common condition seen across the range of household pets.

The symptoms are an abnormal consistency of feces – varying from semi-solid to liquid. Blood, mucus, or undigested food may be passed, or there may be unpleasant smelling gas. Affected pets may need to pass feces more frequently than usual, and may strain to pass the stools.

The causes tend to be:

• Dietary – food allergies, eating too much food, imbalanced diet (too little fiber, too much fat), scavenging, and eating inappropriate food.

• Infections – bacteria (such as *E. coli,* salmonella campylobacter, Tyzzer's disease), viruses (such as canine parvovirus, feline infectious enteritis).

• Pancreatic insufficiency causes long-term diarrhea (see page 132).

• Malabsorption syndrome – if the lining of the bowel has been damaged by infection or some other cause, it may lose the ability to absorb nutrients completely from the food traveling through the intestines. This leads to long-term diarrhea.

• Colitis – a form of acute diarrhea, in which the bowel lining is inflamed, and blood and mucus are passed in the feces, which are loose and watery.

Diarrhea in parrots is often the result of drinking a lot of water as a reaction to stress.

• Parasites – large numbers of bowel parasites will predispose to diarrhea.

• Poisons – lead and mercury will cause diarrhea, amongst other symptoms.

• Tumors – small tumors may irritate and cause diarrhea (large tumors tend to cause obstruction and constipation).

• Gerbils may contract salmonella and occasionally "wet tail," causing diarrhea. Wet tail in hamsters is a common syndrome – watery diarrhea soils the tail area. It is caused by a combination of infective agents triggered by stress.

• Birds are very susceptible to loose and watery droppings as a result of sudden dietary changes, stress, antibiotics, parasites, or infections. Parrots sometimes drink large amounts of water when stressed, this can result in very watery droppings.

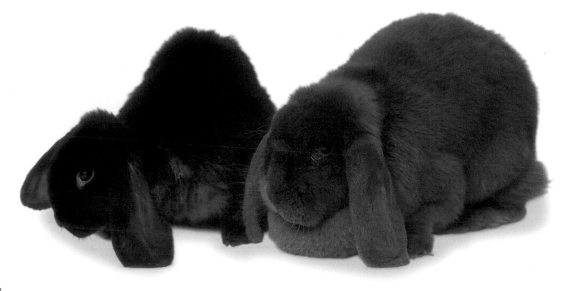

REMEDIES

Treat any underlying specific cause, such as an infection or parasites. Check the pet's diet and adjust it if necessary – this is often the best way of treating non-infective causes of diarrhea. Common sense may be all that is required – to lower fiber content, or decrease fat levels – but veterinary advice may be needed. If you are not sure what change in diet will be helpful, consult your local practice.

NUTRITIONAL

Probiotics will help restore normal balance of beneficial bacteria in the bowel. Live yoghurt will help, but a specific probiotic supplement is usually more beneficial.

AROMATHERAPY

Cinnamon leaf is a good antidiarrhea remedy and helps energize patients debilitated by a bout of diarrhea.
Neroli is good for chronic, persistent diarrhoea, especially if accompanied by flatulence and colic.
Ginger soothes the discomfort and soreness of inflamed bowels.

HERBAL

Meadowsweet – generally upset digestion with diarrhea and flatulence.
Fennel – good for irritable bowels, prone to frequent bouts of diarrhea or colitis, often very gassy bowels.
Liquorice – soothing and calming for inflamed bowels, and for persistent bowel infections. Large doses may be laxative – use carefully.
Peppermint – an effective digestive stabiliser, good for colitis, flatulence, diarrhea, and colic. Very comforting for the stomach.
Ginger – warming and comforting for the digestion. Good for persistent bowel inflammation.
Slippery elm – the best of all the herbal remedies for diarrhea. For all types of diarrhea, relieves inflammation, lines the bowel, and calms and soothes the digestive tract. Suitable for all pets.

HOMEOPATHY

Aloe – diarrhea following overuse of drugs, sudden acute diarrhea with mucus and flatulence.
Arsen. alb. – diarrhea caused by food poisoning, usually with vomiting. Patient is restless and anxious.
Camomile – watery, greenish, frothy diarrhea (often when young animals are teething).
Colchicum – straining, with jelly-like feces.
Colocynth – straining, with arched back and severe colic.
Lycopodium – solid material within a loose stool.
Merc. sol. – thick, pasty diarrhea, not painful, no straining.
Merc. corr. – thinner, spurting diarrhea, some straining and discomfort.
Nux vomica – diarrhea (or constipation) following eating of unsuitable food.
Phosphorus – mucus and blood in feces, often unpleasant smelling; patient becomes weak very quickly.
Podophyllum – "explosive" diarrhea with lots of gas and watery feces.
Pulsatilla – varying from diarrhea to normal feces; never passes two stools alike.
Rhus tox. – straining to pass watery, yellow, frothy, blood-stained stools.
Vervatrum alb. – acute diarrhea; patient feels cold to touch, and may collapse.

BELOW *Ginger is a natural remedy that soothes the discomfort of irritated bowels.*

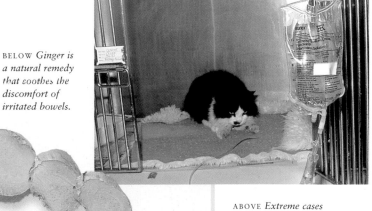

ABOVE *Extreme cases of diarrhea may lead to acute dehydration.*

Urinary incontinence

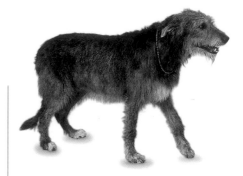

Incontinence can develop as a consequence of aging and resultant muscle weakness.

This is a leaking of urine, which may be occasional and only in small amounts, or frequent and copious.

The symptoms are a dribbling of urine, often when the animal is at rest or asleep; it may be unaware of this.

The causes are either congenital, acquired, or traumatic. If congenital, there is a malformation of the ureter, the tube that carries urine from the bladder to the outside. This is a problem found mainly in bitches. Acquired means that there has been a gradual weakening of the muscle that controls the opening to the bladder, letting urine leak out. This is mainly a problem in middle-aged, neutered bitches. The hormonal change of neutering leads to this weakening. Incontinence can develop as a consequence of aging and generalized muscle weakness. If the cause is traumatic it may follow an accident or injury that has damaged the nerve supply to the bladder. This is often the case when a cat or dog has been hurt in a road accident.

URINARY SYSTEM

The bladder, kidneys, and their connections form the urinary system. This controls fluid balance in the body and gets rid of waste products. If you suspect your pet has a urinary system problem, take a fresh sample of urine in a sterile container when you visit the vet.

REMEDIES

Surgery may be required for congenital ureter problems. Drugs may control acquired incontinence, but often the problem becomes more difficult to control as the patient gets older and the condition tends to deteriorate.

ACUPUNCTURE
Regular acupuncture can improve control with both acquired and traumatic incontinence.

PHYSIOTHERAPY
Exercise and stretching techniques will improve muscular control of the bladder.

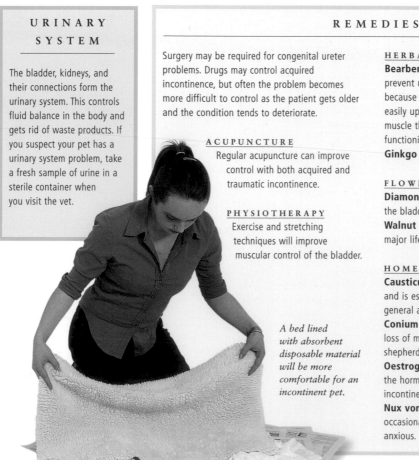

A bed lined with absorbent disposable material will be more comfortable for an incontinent pet.

HERBAL
Bearberry (uva ursi) and **buchu** will help prevent urinary infection, which is a constant risk because of the leakage of urine. Infection tracks easily up into the bladder when the sphincter muscle that normally "seals" the bladder is not functioning properly.
Ginkgo – a tonic remedy to help tone muscles.

FLOWER AND GEM REMEDIES
Diamond and **pearl** gem essences help "tone" the bladder and its sphincter, and improve control.
Walnut – where incontinence occurs after a major life change such as a move of house.

HOMEOPATHY
Causticum – strengthens weak bladder muscles, and is especially helpful in old animals, with general arthritis and muscle weakness.
Conium – for general hind-end weakness and loss of muscle strength, especially in German shepherd dogs with CDRM (see page 120).
Oestrogen – a homeopathic remedy made from the hormone will help bitches with acquired incontinence following neutering.
Nux vomica – for irritable animals that occasionally dribble urine when excited or anxious.

Cystitis

Cystitis is an inflammation of the bladder and more common in females.

The symptoms are frequent urination, straining to pass urine, blood in urine, and pain on passing urine.

The causes are:
• Bacterial infection – infection usually tracks up into the bladder from outside. It is easier for the bacteria to gain access to the bladder in incontinent animals or pets that are in season, or if the bladder has been injured, or if the bladder is not being emptied regularly.
• Trauma – injury to the bladder.
• Bladder stones – stones that are developing in the bladder, some types of which are rough and spiky, will irritate the lining of the bladder, causing cystitis.
• Tumors – bladder tumors cause inflammation as they grow, also causing cystitis.

Cystitis is most common in dogs and cats, but all pets can be affected. Rabbit urine varies considerably in color – it can be clear, yellow, brown, or bright red. The red color is caused by pigments found in plant materials that the rabbit has eaten. Red-colored urine is not necessarily caused by blood in the urine. A urine test may be needed if there is any doubt because rabbits do suffer from cystitis occasionally.

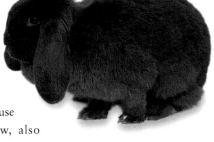

The urine passed by rabbits can vary considerably in color. This is due to pigmentation from plant materials.

CAUSES

• bacterial infection
• trauma
• bladder stones
• tumors

SIGNS AND SYMPTOMS

• frequent urination
• straining to pass urine
• blood in urine
• pain on passing urine

REMEDIES

To treat cystitis, the animal should drink plenty of fluids – make sure mineral water is available.

AROMATHERAPY
Massaging with essential oils is very soothing and comforting for cystitis sufferers.
Bergamot – cystitis accompanied by vaginal infection and discharge.
Lavender – cystitis with anxiety and distress.
Tea tree – treats the infection, relieves soreness.
Sandalwood – cystitis caused by bacterial infection.
Juniper – cystitis with anxiety and tension.
Frankincense – cystitis triggered by stress.
Parsley seed and **celery seed** – all forms of urinary infection.
Yarrow – cystitis accompanied by digestive problems.
Thyme – cystitis following a severe chill.

FLOWER AND GEM REMEDIES
Diamond and **redwood** both relieve symptoms.

HERBAL
Bearberry (uva ursi) and **buchu** – first-line herbal treatments for cystitis.
Marshmallow – irritable bladder accompanied by irritable bowel syndrome.

Juniper – for acute or chronic cystitis.
Kava kava – cystitis with vaginal discharge.
Nettles – for the irritation and discomfort of cystitis.
Saw palmetto – for cystitis in male animals, especially if accompanied by prostate problems.
Damiana – cystitis with weakness and debility.
Cranberry – the juice is a urinary antiseptic.

HOMOEOPATHY
Cantharis is the classic remedy for acute cystitis – burning pain on passing urine, blood in urine, small amounts of urine passed frequently. If given early enough, will almost always cure cystitis symptoms in a matter of hours.
Thlapsi bursa – for chronic cystitis when there is blood in urine, but less acute symptoms than cantharis.

NUTRITIONAL
Vitamin C will help prevent and treat cystitis.

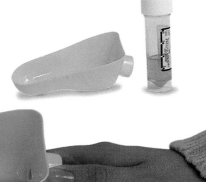

A urine test will establish the presence of urinary problems.

Kidney disease

ACUTE KIDNEY DISEASE

CAUSES

- bacterial or viral infection
- poisoning

SIGNS AND SYMPTOMS

- loss of appetite
- vomiting
- diarrhea or constipation
- rapid weight loss
- increased thirst
- smell of urea on breath
- convulsions

CHRONIC KIDNEY DISEASE

CAUSES

- infections and abscesses in the kidneys
- poisoning
- tumors
- kidney stones
- blockage of urinary tract

SIGNS AND SYMPTOMS

- increased thirst
- increased passing of urine
- vomiting
- smell of urea on breath
- mouth ulcers
- diarrhea
- poor skin and coat condition
- dehydration
- debility
- anemia

Tortoises can be affected by kidney disease.

Kidney disease, or renal failure, is a common condition of older animals, especially cats, and may be acute or chronic.

The symptoms of acute kidney disease are loss of appetite, vomiting, diarrhea or constipation, rapid weight loss, increased thirst, not passing urine, smell of urea on breath, and convulsions. The symptoms of chronic kidney disease are increased thirst, passing much more urine, vomiting, smell of urea on breath, mouth ulcers, diarrhea, poor skin and coat condition, dehydration, debility, and anemia.

Anemia occurs because the kidneys fail to produce a hormone called erythropoetin, which is needed in the manufacture of red blood cells. Weight loss results from the kidneys failure to filter and retain proteins and other body nutrients.

The causes of acute kidney disease are bacterial or viral infections and poisons.

The causes of chronic kidney disease are infections and abscesses in the kidneys, toxins and poisons carried via the bloodstream to the kidneys, kidney tumors, and kidney stones. Blockage of the urinary tract, such as by a bladder stone, can also cause kidney damage.

- Most kidney problems are in dogs and cats. A large proportion of older cats suffer some degree of chronic kidney disease. Thyroid disease causes similar symptoms to kidney disease, so not all thirsty old cats with weight loss have kidney disease!
- Tortoises may be affected by kidney disease. This shows as gradual weight loss over several months, sometimes with swelling of the legs. Kidney disease in tortoises is mainly caused by an infection with a protozoal organism.

Acute kidney disease is life-threatening and requires immediate veterinary treatment. Intravenous drugs and other emergency support treatment will be necessary. Underlying problems such as infections need to be treated. Natural medicines are effective, particularly in supporting chronic failing kidneys. Treat acute kidney failure with natural remedies for shock and collapse (see page 182).

AROMATHERAPY
Yarrow – for kidney infections, acute or chronic.
Bergamot – for chronic kidney failure, with mouth ulcers.
Lavender – for pain and discomfort over the kidneys.
Cajeput – for infections that track up to the kidneys.
Nutmeg – for all bacterial infections.
Parsley seed and **celery seed** – for infection throughout the urinary tract.
Tea tree – for kidney infections.

FLOWER AND GEM REMEDIES
Olive – for the weakness and debility of kidney disease.
Pearl – for all forms of kidney disease.
Dill – for kidney stones: helps the body dissolve them.
Redwood – for chronic renal failure.

HERBAL
Bearberry – use regularly for pets with chronic kidney failure.
Buchu – a useful support remedy for chronic kidney disease.
Cayenne – improves circulation to the kidneys, so stimulates healing in kidney disease.
Nettles – increase throughput to the kidneys, so helping to flush toxins out of the kidneys.

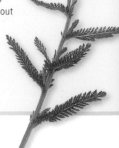

Yarrow treats both acute and chronic kidney infections.

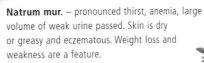

REMEDIES

CRYSTAL AND GEM ESSENCES

Amber – detoxifying, good for chronic kidney function.
Jade – for kidney disease with retained fluid.
Pearl – for all forms of kidney disease.

HOMEOPATHY

Arsen. alb. – chronic kidney disease, with increased thirst, but for small amounts of water little and often. Patient is very restless and anxious, need for warmth. A dry skin with dandruff. Symptoms worse toward the middle of the night.
Berberis – kidney disease is often accompanied by liver disease. Urine output may alternate between being much more than usual, then much less than usual. Discomfort and weakness over the lower back, pelvis, and over the kidneys.
Eel serum – sudden onset kidney failure, when urine stops being produced. In these cases, Eel serum will help get the urine moving again, and promote fluid production by the kidneys.
Kali chlor. – for acute or chronic kidney disease, often blood and protein passed in urine. Good for mouth ulceration, especially in chronic kidney disease in cats. Vomiting is a common symptom, as is a greenish diarrhea.
Merc. corr. – chronic kidney disorders with blood in urine. Often associated with bowel inflammation leading to diarrhea. Patient tends to have a wet mouth because of excessive salivation.
Merc. sol. – much salivation, mouth ulcers, and spongy gums, increased thirst. Urine may be dark in color.

Kidney disease will cause a noticeable increase in thirst.

Natrum mur. – pronounced thirst, anemia, large volume of weak urine passed. Skin is dry or greasy and eczematous. Weight loss and weakness are a feature.
Phosphorus – kidney disease with brown or red sediment being passed in the urine. Suits thin, nervous patients, with rapid onset of symptoms.
Plumbum met. – chronic degenerative kidney failure, dry skin, weak heart and circulation.
Urtica – for acute renal failure, helps stimulate fluid flow through the kidneys.

NUTRITIONAL

Vitamins will help boost the normal functioning of the kidneys. A multivitamin supplement will be beneficial. **Vitamin B-complex** is the most useful vitamin to help ailing kidneys.

ABOVE *Kidney disease is more commonly found in older animals, especially cats.*

BELOW *Olive will help with the general weakness and debility of kidney disease.*

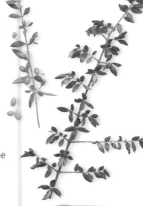

Urinary stones (urolithiasis)

CAUSES

- bacterial infection
- congenital abnormality
- liver disease
- insufficient water intake
- acid or alkaline imbalance in urine

SIGNS AND SYMPTOMS

- difficulty in passing urine
- pain on passing urine
- blood in urine
- arching of the back

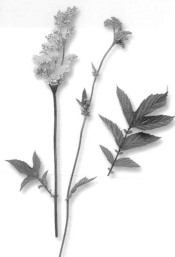

ABOVE *The action of meadowsweet is to dissolve fine, sandy mineral deposits.*

BELOW *Kidney stones, called uroliths, can vary in size from tiny crystals to large stones.*

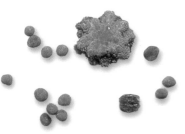

Uroliths or calculi are the names used to describe stones made up of minerals, which form in the bladder or occasionally in the kidneys or urethra – the tube that drains urine from the bladder to the outside. These can vary in size from tiny crystals, too small to be seen with the naked eye, to visible sediment, "gravel" in the urine, or large stones that may become too large to be passed and so stay in the bladder. These may cause an obstruction.

The symptoms are a difficulty in passing urine, pain on passing urine, blood in the urine, arching of the back, or passing small quantities of urine very frequently. If complete obstruction occurs, there is severe pain, with no urine passed and the abdomen swelling as the bladder becomes enlarged.

Different types of uroliths can form. Various minerals are present, dissolved in the urine, at all times. Bacteria may predispose these minerals in the urine to settle out and form crystals. Dietary factors also may predispose to crystal formation. Cats with struvite crystal problems are described as having FLUTD (feline lower urinary tract disease), which is also known as FUS (feline urological syndrome).

Dogs may form six main kinds of uroliths: struvite, urate, cystine, phosphate, oxalate, and silicate. Phosphate calculi are the most common – these are probably associated with bacterial infection, the bacteria acting as a focus for the minerals to crystallize around. Cystine calculi are usually formed because of a genetic defect that lets excess cystine be passed via the kidneys into the urine. Urate calculi are formed either as a result of liver disease, which can produce excess urates in the urine, or as a result of a genetic defect in the dalmatian breed.

Other factors affect the likelihood of uroliths forming. Too little water intake will be a major factor in allowing minerals in solution to crystallize – the more an animal drinks, the more dilute the urine will be, the more urine is passed, and the less the chance of crystals being formed.

The acidity or alkalinity of the urine is another predisposing cause. Struvite crystals, for instance, are much less likely to occur in a slightly acidic urine, whereas oxalate and urate are much more likely to form in an acidic urine. Cystine crystallizes out more easily at a neutral pH (pH is the measure of how acid or alkaline the urine is).

Some stones cause more physical damage to the bladder than others. For instance, oxalate stones are rough and spiky, cystine are smooth. In severe cases of urolithiasis where a blockage has occurred, or where there are a large numbers of sizeable stones, or one or two very large stones, surgery is essential. If any pet is straining to pass urine, and cannot do so, emergency veterinary treatment is necessary. Apart from treating any underlying problems, such as cystitis or infection, the urine should be made more (or less) acid or alkaline, depending on the type of stone present – by adding acidifying agents or alkalizing agents to the diet. Veterinary expertise is essential to be able to find out which level of acidity or alkalinity is required.

AROMATHERAPY

Juniper helps all bladder problems, including sediment in the urine.
Tea tree helps keep infection at bay.

Juniper is a useful remedy for all bladder problems.

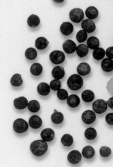

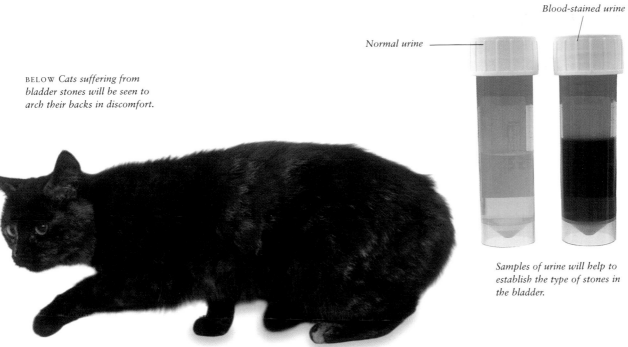

Blood-stained urine

Normal urine

BELOW *Cats suffering from bladder stones will be seen to arch their backs in discomfort.*

Samples of urine will help to establish the type of stones in the bladder.

REMEDIES

FLOWER AND GEM-PEARL REMEDIES
Pearl and **dill** relieve the bladder irritation caused by crystal formation.

HERBAL
Bearberry (uva ursi) helps dissolve bladder stones and gravel.
Meadow sweet – useful to dissolve fine sandy mineral deposits.
Nettles and **parsley piert** – help flush fine sand and stones from the bladder.
Couchgrass and **birch leaves** – relieve bladder inflammation caused by calculi.

Pearl will help relieve bladder irritation.

HOMEOPATHY
Thlaspi bursa – good for chronic cystitis especially in cats with FUS (FLUTD). It helps dissolve crystals, reduces inflammation, and flushes through fine crystals.
Benzoic acid – a good remedy for urolithiasis, where the urine being produced is dark in color and slightly sweet-smelling.
Calc. carb. – for overweight, big boned animals,

usually with small numbers of larger stones.
Lycopodium – if reddish brown, sandy material is being passed in the urine.
Sarsaparilla – for thick, mucoid material formed, which may cause an obstruction.

NUTRITIONAL
Appropriate acidifying or alkalizing agents. For instance, **vitamin C** helps to acidify the urine, as well as helping the bladder wall to heal, where it has been damaged by the crystals or stones. Vitamin C also helps fight infection in the urine, which predisposes to the formation of stones.
Sodium bicarbonate is a good alkalizing agent. Check with your veterinarian to find out which kind of uroliths are present, and whether the urine needs to be more acid or alkaline.
Cranberry juice – will relieve the inflammation caused by the calculi.
Increasing or restricting certain minerals will help reduce the formation of new stones. For instance, cats with FUS will have a lower chance of re-formation of stones if magnesium is restricted in the diet.
Check with your veterinarian on which minerals or other constituents of the diet should be altered to help control the problem.

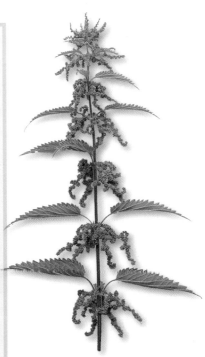

Nettles will help to flush away any fine sediment that forms in the bladder.

Uterus (womb) disease

Uterine infection can occur after giving birth and may become an acute condition.

Uterine disease is most commonly an inflammation or infection of the lining of the womb.

The symptoms are bloodstained or purulent discharge from the vagina (although in some cases of uterine disease there is no visible outward discharge, because the disease is sealed within the womb), increased thirst, poor appetite, intermittent vomiting, a high temperature (in acute cases of infection), and abdominal swelling if a large volume of pus forms in the uterus.

The causes are: bacterial infection, often occurring just after giving birth; accumulation of uterine secretions, often occurring soon after being in season; and uterine cancer – usually no discharge. Acute infection occurring just after birth is known as metritis, and can be life-threatening; immediate veterinary treatment is necessary if this occurs.

The accumulation of secretions in the uterus is a condition known as pyometra, and is particularly common in unneutered bitches as they get older. It occurs occasionally in ferrets and cats, but is rarely found in other pets.

A pet with serious metritis or pyometra will need immediate veterinary treatment, which may necessitate surgery to remove the enlarged womb in the case of pyometra.

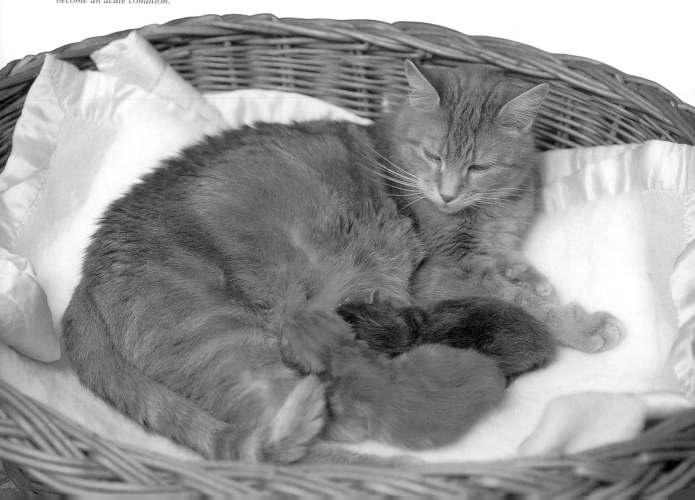

REMEDIES

Natural medicines are invaluable in both acute and chronic uterine disease, and may avoid the necessity of surgery if used in the early stages of pyometra. Because of the potentially serious nature of these problems, natural medicines should be used only under the direction of a veterinarian with the appropriate expertise.

AROMATHERAPY

Tea tree and **lemon eucalyptus** are good anti-infective agents for uterine infections.
Jasmine or **lavender** relieve inflammation and reduce secretions in the uterus.

HERBAL

Motherwort – good for most uterine disorders, especially following hormonal change, such as uterine infection occurring after being in season.
Raspberry – tones the uterus, and helps expel retained discharges.

CRYSTAL AND GEM ESSENCES

Hematite – for uterine problems with major loss of bloodstained discharge.
Moonstone – for uterine infection which is accompanied by vaginal discharge.
Unakite – suitable for all diseases of the reproductive system.

HOMEOPATHY

Caulophyllum – for chocolate-colored, runny discharge from the vagina.
Belladonna – for acute metritis with high fever.
Helonias – chronic infection or inflammation of the uterus, with tenderness on pressure over the lower back.

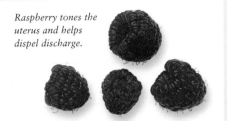

Raspberry tones the uterus and helps dispel discharge.

Ferrum. phos. – early stages of uterine infection, especially if bloodstained discharge is passed.
Hydrastis – for early pyometra, with catarrhal or purulent discharge from womb. Discharge is usually thick and yellow in color.
Hepar. sulph. – the classic homeopathic remedy to fight pus formation.
Sabina – large amounts of fresh blood being passed from the uterus, especially in the case of pyometra.
Sepia – for chronic, persistent, uterine infection and discharges, weakness at the base of the tail.
Secale – dark blood and foul-smelling discharge from the vagina.

TEMPERATURES

The normal temperature of dogs and cats is 101.5°F (38.5°C). A temperature of 102.5°F (39.3°C) and above is abnormal. A temperature of 104°F (40°C) is serious and needs immediate veterinary attention.

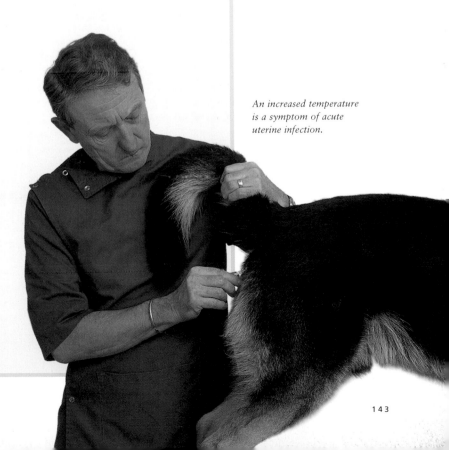

An increased temperature is a symptom of acute uterine infection.

Eucalyptus is an anti-infective agent for uterine diseases.

Infertility

CAUSES

- infection
- problems in uterus, ovaries or fallopian tubes: obstructions, scarring, thickened wall, cysts
- hormonal imbalance
- obesity
- poor diet

There are many and varied causes of infertility in pets. Obesity and hormone imbalance are common causes.

Generally, small pets such as gerbils, guinea pigs, and rabbits have a low incidence of infertility, whereas cats, and even more so, bitches are more often affected.

The causes are many and varied, but often unknown. They may include any of the following:

- Infection in vagina and uterus.
- Obstructions and scarring in uterus or fallopian tubes.
- Hormone imbalance, preventing egg production, or implantation of the embryo into the uterus. This may be caused by imbalance in female, or thyroid hormones.
- Thickened wall of uterus – preventing implanting of embryo.
- Obesity.
- Poor diet – good nutrition is required for pregnancy to occur. Cats will become infertile if there is insufficient taurine in the diet.

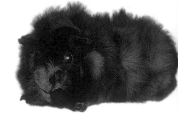

Guinea pigs generally have a low incidence of infertility.

- Ferrets can stay in season for long periods if unmated and the excess estrogen (female hormone) produced can damage bone marrow, which leads to anemia. Affected ferrets lose weight and fur, have difficulty breathing, and are very pale.
- Old female gerbils may develop cystic ovaries. These cause infertility – although affected gerbils often look pregnant because of the greatly enlarged ovaries.
- Problems in the male pet may cause apparent infertility in the female. If in doubt, use other males for breeding.

Cats, like ferrets, tend to stay on heat until they are mated. This can be debilitating, as well as a difficult problem to contend with for their owners. It is very hard to keep track of a cat that for long periods of time is trying to escape and find a partner.

REMEDIES

For treatment, ensure a good basic diet.

AROMATHERAPY
Celery seed stimulates correct glandular secretion, including production of eggs from the ovaries.

HERBAL
Motherwort – balances hormones to improve fertility.
Raspberry leaf – tones the uterus to aid implantation of embryo.

FLOWER AND GEM REMEDIES
Clematis – where the female lacks interest in the male.
Larch – where the female is shy, lacking in confidence, and anxious.

CRYSTAL AND GEM ESSENCES
Moonstone – stimulates a balanced hormone secretion to aid fertility.
Unakite – where fertility has been affected by infections of the reproductive tract, or by administration of drugs.

Moonstone

HOMEOPATHY
Iodum – in thin females, active, restless, but not coming in season regularly.
Lachesis – jealous, suspicious individuals. Produce very dark red or purple blood when in season; mammary glands may have a purple discoloration.
Lilium tig. – restless, anxious types, appear

to be hurried and worried. Prefer not to be fussed over, and often seem to want to be on their own.
Murex – repeated "calling" (being on heat) in female cats, but don't actually get pregnant easily.
Sepia – moody females; sometimes aggressive if handled too much.
Pulsatilla – shy, gentle, quiet females; like contact and affection, but can have mood swings.

NUTRITIONAL
Vitamin E, **selenium** and **vitamin B-complex** all help maintain fertility. A good balanced, nutritious diet – as close to the natural diet as possible is necessary to be healthy and fertile.

False pregnancy

This is a set of symptoms which imitate the physical changes that occur during pregnancy. It is a condition mainly seen in bitches and sometimes in rabbits.

The symptoms differ according to time. Approximately three weeks after the end of the season, there is a loss of energy, increase in appetite, and swelling of the abdomen. At the time or shortly before the bitch would be giving birth (six to nine weeks after a season), she is likely to be nest-making, anxious and whining, and producing milk in the mammary glands.

The reasons for the development of false pregnancies is not fully understood, but is presumed to be a hormonal imbalance. In the wild, most bitches would become pregnant after a season, so the body's hormonal system is geared up to be pregnant. In a sense, not being pregnant is the abnormal state, so it is natural for the

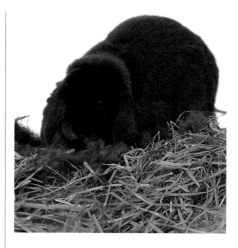

Rabbits are also prone to false pregnancy. An obvious symptom is nest-making.

hormones to produce the changes in the reproductive system that would occur in a "truly" pregnant animal.

Rabbits are the only other pet in which "imaginary" pregnancies are regularly seen. This is mainly in the form of nest-making.

CAUSES

- not fully understood, but presumed to be a hormonal imbalance

SIGNS AND SYMPTOMS

three weeks after end of season:
- loss of energy
- increased appetite
- swelling of the abdomen

six to nine weeks after end of season:
- nest-making
- anxiety
- whining
- production of milk in mammary glands

REMEDIES

In mild cases, symptoms of false pregnancy resolve naturally in a short time and no treatment is necessary. In more severe cases, bitches can be dull and depressed and produce large amounts of milk, which predisposes to mastitis. Symptoms can last for many weeks, and may become more intense after each successive season. Conventional treatment usually involves giving hormonal drugs, which often have side-effects, and are not always particularly effective. Neutering of bitches prone to false pregnancies is also often advised. Natural therapies are frequently very effective.

HERBAL
Raspberry leaf – ideal to use as preventive; start giving as soon as the season ends, or as treatment during a false pregnancy.

CRYSTAL AND GEM ESSENCES
Moonstone – balances hormones and reduces tendency for false pregnancy to occur.

HOMEOPATHY
Sepia – for bitches that become moody, morose, and snappy, and want to be left alone during a false pregnancy.
Pulsatilla – for bitches that are shy, gentle, and variable in their moods, and may produce a lot of milk.
Bryonia – helps dry up the milk in hard, swollen glands.
Cyclamen – dries up milk when the mammary glands are "dripping" with milk.

Raspberry leaf can be given as a preventative treatment to avoid false pregnancy.

DOS AND DON'TS

Do reduce the water intake considerably for a couple of days. This will help to minimize milk production, as will cutting down the carbohydrate content of the diet.

Do increase the exercise given. This will help physically to minimize symptoms, but will also to distract the bitch from the mental and emotional symptoms.

Don't have a bitch neutered during a false pregnancy – this can cause symptoms to persist.

Mastitis

CAUSES

- bacterial infection
- mammary cancer

SIGNS AND SYMPTOMS

- hot, swollen, painful mammary glands
- abscess
- high temperature
- lethargy
- decreased appetite

This is an inflammation, usually caused by an infection, in one or more mammary glands.

The symptoms are hot, swollen, painful mammary glands. An abscess may form, which will eventually burst, with a large amount of foul pus discharging from it. The affected pet will run a high temperature, be lethargic, and will eat less than usual.

It is usually caused by a bacterial infection, which often affects the glands just after birth, during a false pregnancy, or when there is mammary cancer present.

Guinea pigs are prone to mastitis, especially if their environment is unhygienic – cages that are poorly cleaned; food and water not changed frequently. Rabbits are often affected at the time of weaning, especially if this is carried out very suddenly, and earlier than usual (at 3 or 4 weeks rather than 7 or 8 weeks after giving birth).

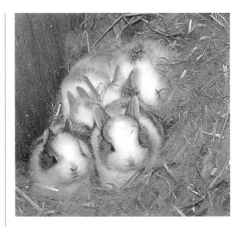

Rabbits can be affected by mastitis if they are weaned suddenly and earlier than usual.

The mammary glands on all pets will be swollen and warm when they are lactating. These normal symptoms should not be confused with the hard, hot, painful swelling of mastitis – if in any doubt, always consult your veterinarian.

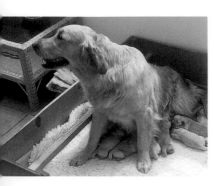

Mastitis is often caused by bacterial infection after birth.

REMEDIES

Conventional treatment in severe cases of mastitis is usually antibiotics against the infection.

AROMATHERAPY
Celery seed and **dill seed** will increase milk flow, helping to flush out toxins from infected mammary glands. Don't massage directly into glands – use around the glands oradminister by diffusion.
Lavender – soothes and heals inflamed mammary tissue.

Lavender will soothe and heal inflamed mammary tissue.

HERBAL
Aloe vera – use externally as a gel to relieve soreness and heal ulcerated mammary glands. Ulceration easily develops when the glands are tense and swollen.

HOMEOPATHY
Belladonna – for swollen glands with acute fever.
Bryonia – for hot, solid, hard glands where the discomfort is less when at rest, but worse when the patient gets up and moves about.
Phytolacca – for firm, nodular glands.
Hepar sulph. – when abscessation is present.
Silicea – use after symptoms have subsided, to minimize thickening and scarring of the glands.

NUTRITIONAL
Vitamin C helps fight infection in the glands and promotes healing of damaged tissue.
Malt and **crushed onion** applied to the glands as a salve, to soothe and reduce swelling. Do not apply to broken or ulcerated skin.

Abortion/resorption

There are two main problems that can happen during pregnancy – death of the fetus (and their abortion or resorption), and pregnancy toxemia of the mother.

In the case of abortion/resorption, when one or more fetuses die in the womb, they are normally expelled (abortion) or resorbed back into the body of the mother (resorption). The later the stage of pregnancy, the more likely abortion is to occur; whereas in the first week or two of pregnancy, resorption is more likely.

In resorption, there are no obvious symptoms except that the pregnancy does not continue. In some cases, the pregnancy may not be known – and in some cases of infertility, it may be that the female becomes pregnant, but early resorption takes place.

Accidents and injuries can cause abortion or resorption, as can viruses, bacteria, and poor nutrition.

REMEDIES

NUTRITIONAL
Vitamin E will help prevent abortion/resorption, as will any good multivitamin or mineral supplement.

HOMEOPATHY
Viburnum opulis – very effective in combating early abortion or resorption.
Cobaltum nitricum – useful for those females where repeated abortion occurs.
Kali carb – an effective remedy to help return females back to full health.

HERBAL
Raspberry leaf, like **caullophyllum,** strengthens and tones the uterus muscles, minimizes the risk of abortion, and reduces the likelihood of problems during birth.
Caulophyllum given during the later stages of pregnancy will help to tone the uterus, reduce the likelihood of abortion, and prepare the uterus for an easy birth.

CAUSES
- not fully understood, but presumed to be a hormonal imbalance

SIGNS AND SYMPTOMS
- abortion or resorption of fetus(es)

DOS AND DON'TS
Don't discourage normal exercise in pregnant pets.

Do keep aborted fetus for examination.

Pregnancy toxemia

This is a condition seen late in pregnancy, where toxins build-up in the body, causing severe illness or death.

The symptoms are lethargy, weakness, collapse, difficulty in breathing, and rapid onset of coma, followed by death.

The causes are not fully understood. Affected animals that die often show signs of liver failure and fatty degeneration of the liver. Nutritional imbalance may be a trigger factor where some individuals cannot cope with the strain put on the distribution and absorption of nutrients. It is a life-threatening emergency that requires immediate veterinary treatment.

REMEDIES

FLOWER AND GEM REMEDIES
Rescue Remedy will alleviate the shock.

HOMEOPATHY
Aconite – for collapse in acute cases.
Lycopodium – for the metabolic and nutritional imbalance that is thought to underlie the onset of pregnancy toxemia.
Phosphorus for the rapid destruction of liver and other organs, which occurs in pregnancy toxemia.
Calc. phos. – give throughout pregnancy to pets that have previously had pregnancy toxemia to help prevent it recurring.

CAUSES
- not fully understood – may be liver failure

SIGNS AND SYMPTOMS
- lethargy
- weakness
- collapse
- diffiluty in breathing
- rapid onset of coma or death

Egg-binding

CAUSES

- nutritional imbalance
- hormonal imbalance

SIGNS AND SYMPTOMS

- dullness/depression
- blood or mucus passed when straining to pass the egg

Species of pets that lay eggs – birds, lizards, snakes, tortoises, and terrapins – may develop egg-binding. In this condition, as the name suggests, eggs that are meant to be laid remain stuck, or bound, in the uterus.

A dull, depressed pet is likely to be suffering from this condition. When straining to pass the egg, it may pass blood or mucus.

It has nutritional and hormonal causes. Nutritionally, it is a mineral imbalance; hormonally, there are insufficient hormones to stimulate the muscular contractions to push the eggs out.

- In tortoises and terrapins, the lack of a suitable site for egg-laying prevents the female from laying her eggs, and the uterus "closes down" so that the egg is not released.
- In lizards, egg-binding is usually caused by calcium deficiency, kidney disease, or an inappropriate environment.

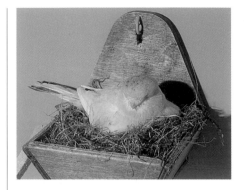

ABOVE *Species that lay eggs sometimes develop egg-binding.*

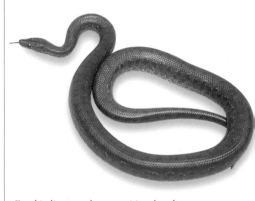

Egg-binding may have nutritional and hormonal causes.

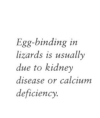

Egg-binding in lizards is usually due to kidney disease or calcium deficiency.

REMEDIES

As far as treatment is concerned, surgery to remove eggs may be required in some cases. In hormonal "inertia" of the uterus, use the remedies for Problems giving birth (see opposite), especially **Caulophyllum**. If nutritional/metabolic factors are the cause, extra **calcium** may be needed, and homeopathic **Calc. phos.** will be beneficial. If infection is a cause, use homeopathic **Hepar. sulph.** In all cases, use remedies for bruising, as the internal tissues will be damaged and sore.

HOMEOPATHY
Arnica and **bellis** per. are ideal.

Problems giving birth

Dystocia is the term used to describe difficulty with giving birth. There are three main reasons for dystocia: uterine inertia, a failure of the uterus to contract and push the fetuses out of the body; oversized fetus, when the fetus is simply too large to pass through the birth canal; and wrongly positioned fetus, which cannot leave in the head-first position.

The symptoms to look for are persistent straining, with no fetuses born, eventually lack of straining, and dull, lethargic mother. In species that have several fetuses, dystocia may mean that no fetuses are born, or that the first few are born safely, but the remainder are unable to be passed.

Uterine inertia can be caused by hormone imbalance, calcium deficiency, and sheer physical tiredness. Anxiety and stress can also cause inertia.

Oversized fetuses are often caused by using a large male to mate a small female. Also, the fetuses of pets that normally give birth to several young will – if there are only one or two fetuses in the womb – be more likely to grow larger than average. Wrongly positioned fetuses seem to occur from time to time without reason.

Although the birth process can take some time, most pets do not stay in labor for long periods. Small pets rarely have problems giving birth, and normally produce their offspring in minutes rather than hours. Dogs and cats take longer, but still only three to four hours in most cases.

Small breeds of dogs, especially short-nosed breeds, are more likely to suffer problems in giving birth. Nervous, anxious, easily stressed bitches are the group most likely to have difficulty.

CAUSES

- uterine inertia
- oversized fetus
- wrongly positioned fetus

SIGNS AND SYMPTOMS

- initially, persistent straining with no fetuses born; later lack of straining and dull, lethargic mother

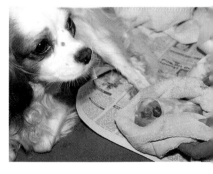

ABOVE *Small breeds of dog are more likely to suffer problems giving birth.*

REMEDIES

In cases of severe dystocia, a cesarian operation may need to be performed to save the lives of both mother and babies. Natural therapies are very effective in cases of uterine inertia.

HERBAL
Raspberry leaf given throughout pregnancy will tone the uterine muscles and facilitate an easy birth.
Motherwort given in the last few days of pregnancy also strengthens the contractions of the uterus, enabling the fetuses to be born easily and quickly.

AROMATHERAPY
Parsley seed used in a diffuser, will help promote normal contractions.

CRYSTAL AND GEM ESSENCES
Jade – during the birth itself. Jade will enhance the power of the uterine muscles and speed up delivery.

HOMEOPATHY
Caulophyllum – the classic homeopathic remedy for an easy birth. Give for the last two-thirds of pregnancy, and give every few minutes during birth, if it seems uterine inertia is setting in.
Arnica – given just after birth will reduce bruising, swelling, and soreness of tissues involved in giving birth.
Bellis per. – use if deep muscular bruising is suspected.

OTHERS
Taking your pet for a ride in a car is a good method of getting the uterus moving when in a state of inertia.

Jade enhances the action of the uterine muscles and helps to speed up delivery.

ABOVE *Raspberry leaf may be given throughout pregnancy to tone the uterine muscles.*

Problems after giving birth

- hormonal imbalance
- stress
- mastitis

SIGNS AND SYMPTOMS

- no milk visible in mammary glands
- hungry, noisy, and distressed offspring

Two main conditions may occur in the female soon after giving birth. One is agalactia – a lack of milk production in the mammary glands. The other is eclampsia – a serious metabolic imbalance associated with producing large amounts of milk.

AGALACTIA

Symptoms of agalactia are hungry, noisy, and distressed offspring and no milk visible in mammary glands.

This condition is caused by hormonal imbalance, stress, or mastitis. It is more commonly found in pets giving birth for the first time.

ECLAMPSIA

Eclampsia is a serious and potentially life-theatening condition. Its symptoms are restlessness, anxiety, high temperature, panting, muscle tremors and spasms, and, eventually, convulsions.

Caused by an imbalance in the supply and mobilization of calcium or glucose within the body. It is mostly seen in dogs with larger than average litters of puppies where the strain from producing large volumes of milk predisposes to eclampsia.

Although eclampsia usually occurs in the bitch soon after birth, the condition can develop in some cases just before birth.

REMEDIES: AGALACTIA

It can be treated in the following ways:

HERBAL
There are several herbs that stimulate milk production in the mammary glands – **milk thistle** and **milkwort** are effective at increasing milk flow.

Fennel and **marshmallow** are also useful in stimulating milk production. Greenleaf herbs, such as **dandelion**, **nettles**, and **parsley**, all have a slightly diuretic effect – they stimulate fluid to be pushed out of the body. One route out is via the mammary glands, and this encourages milk to be produced.

FLOWER AND GEM REMEDIES
Rescue Remedy can help relieve the acute stress and distress of a pet unable to feed her own babies.

HOMEOPATHY
Urtica stimulates milk production, as do **Calc. carb.**, **Calc. phos.**, and **Lecithin**. **Conium** and **iodum** will help if the problem is caused by an under-development of the mammary gland.

OTHERS
Relieve stress as much as possible. Ensure the mother has a safe, secure place to stay with the puppies, away from too many visitors.

Fennel is useful in stimulating milk production.

Eclampsia is more common in breeds that produce large litters.

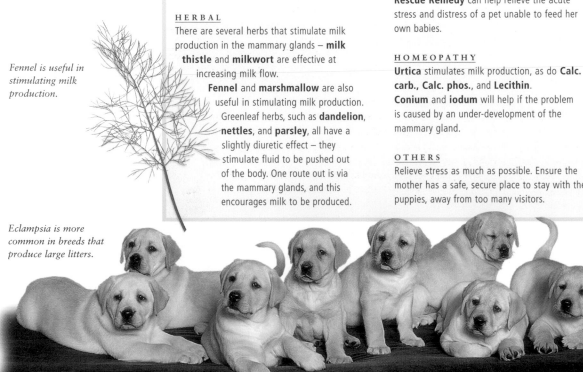

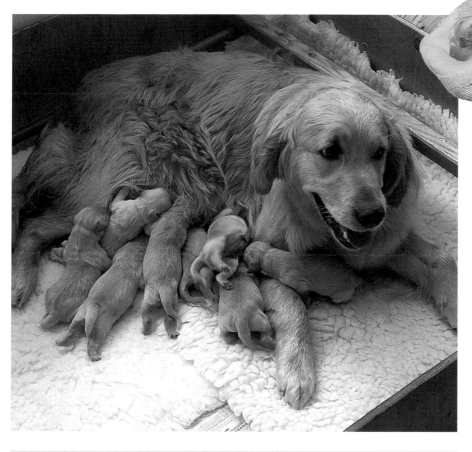

ABOVE *When agalactia has occurred, the puppies get very hungry and may become distressed.*

LEFT *Agalactia is a condition where milk flow ceases. Caused by hormonal imbalance or stress, usually with first litters.*

REMEDIES: ECLAMPSIA

To treat it, intravenous injections of **calcium** are required in all but the mildest of cases. In addition, natural therapies are very effective in speeding up a return to normality and helping to prevent recurrence.

AROMATHERAPY

Lavender is calming and soothing for the hysterical state some bitches exhibit.

FLOWER AND GEM REMEDIES

Rescue Remedy will minimize the shock, distress, and anxiety that is present.

Belladonna will help in reducing fever and the likelihood of convulsions.

HOMEOPATHY

Calc. carb. (for the bigger-framed) and **calc. phos.** (for the smaller, lighter individual) are good preventive remedies for bitches prone to eclampsia.

Arsen. alb. – for the restlessness and anxiety.

Belladonna – for the fever and for convulsions.

Mag. phos. – for the muscle spasms that are part of the symptoms.

Ignatia – for the tension and the emotional stress.

Hyosycamus – for muscle twitching.

Zinc – for weak, trembling, twitching muscles.

ECLAMPSIA

CAUSES

- imbalance in supply and mobilization of calcium or glucose in the body

SIGNS AND SYMPTOMS

- restlessness
- anxiety
- high temperature
- panting
- muscle tremors, spasms, convulsions

Prostate gland disease

The prostate gland is situated near the entrance to the bladder and below the rectum. It has an important secretory function to help keep the male reproductive tract in good working order. Three main conditions can affect the prostate: prostate hyperplasia; prostatitis; and prostate cancer.

The symptoms in all three conditions are similar, since the main effect of each disease is to cause an enlargement and inflammation of the gland. These symptoms are: constipation, or passing flat, ribbon-like feces (caused by upward pressure on the bowel); difficulty in passing urine, passing small amounts of urine frequently, pain on passing urine (caused by pressure on the bladder); blood passed in urine; arched back, abdominal pain; high temperature; loss of appetite, vomiting (if infection is present). Many older pets (like many older men) have a degree of prostate enlargement with age, but symptoms may be minor.

The cause of prostate hyperplasia is a general enlargement and thickening of the prostate. This is due mainly to age and hormonal changes.

Prostatitis, an infection of the prostate, is usually caused by a bladder infection that tracks up into the prostate. Prostatic cancer is a serious, life-threatening tumor that needs specialist treatment.

REMEDIES

There is no specific conventional treatment for prostate cancer. However, any infection should be treated with antibacterial agents. The treatment often advised for prostate hyperplasia is castration. This may seem drastic, but removing testosterone, the male hormone secreted by the testicles, does effectively shrink an enlarged prostate. Natural remedies can often avoid the need for surgery.

HERBAL

Buchu – useful for enlarged prostates, with bladder weakness and incontinence.
Kava kava – good male reproductive remedy for bladder and prostate conditions of all kinds.
Saw palmetto – classic herbal remedy for enlarged prostates, also general strengthening remedy for the debility caused by prostate gland disease.
Damiana – relieves not just prostate disease, butalso the constipation, weakness, and lack of appetite that often accompanies it.

HOMEOPATHY

Baryta carb. – for prostate problems in young dogs that pass urine in a slow stream.

Clematis – for young dogs, with intermittent spurts of urine.
Acid nit. – severely inflamed prostate with blood passed from penis, or in urine.
Cantharis – painful, enlarged prostate; pain and difficulty when passing urine.
Thuja – when there are problems in passing feces because of enlarged prostate.
Ferrum picricum – good for prostate enlargement in the older dog.

NUTRITIONAL

Pumpkin seeds added to the diet help control prostate disease.
Dogs with prostate problems often have an aggravation of symptoms when there is a bitch on heat in the neighborhood. This can happen even (or particularly) in very old dogs.

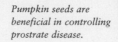

Pumpkin seeds are beneficial in controlling prostrate disease.

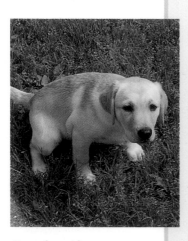

Young dogs with prostate problems often pass urine very slowly.

Orchitis and testicular cancer

These are the two main problems that can affect the testicles.

ORCHITIS

Orchitis is an acute inflammation of one or both testicles. It is not a common condition. The symptoms are a painful, swollen testicle, perhaps with loss of appetite and difficulty in passing urine. The affected pet will be uncomfortable and keep licking at the testicle.

It is caused by injuries and infections – the infection normally entering the testicle through a wound. Any infection in the testicle should be treated.

TESTICULAR CANCER

Several types of testicular cancer occur in pets. Some are slow-growing and do not tend to spread, some are rapidly growing and spread to other organs, and some can cause hormonal changes in the body.

Symptoms to look out for are an enlargement of a testicle (usually only one, and the other testicle may actually become smaller).

As with most cancers, the cause of testicular cancer is not usually known. Male pets retaining one or both testicles inside the abdomen, rather than the testicles moving from the abdomen to their normal position outside the body before or after birth, are far more likely to develop cancer of the testicles as they develop. This is especially true of dogs – it is advisable to discuss with your veterinary practice whether removal of the retained testicle should be undertaken.

One form of testicular cancer in dogs causes a hormonal imbalance and the release of female-like hormones, with the result that the affected dog is "feminised."

REMEDIES: ORCHITIS

AROMATHERAPY
Lavender massaged around the testicles will be calming, and reduce the tendency to lick at the area.

HERBAL
Aloe vera applied in a gel to the testicle will soothe and relieve soreness.

HOMEOPATHY
Belladonna – for hot, lumpy testicles when the acute phase of orchitis has lessened; discomfort is worse when the patient is moving, better at rest.
Rhododendron – scarring of testicles following orchitis.
Arnica – for wounds, bruising, and other injuries to testicles.
Aconite – for inflamed testicles, when the symptoms very first occur.

OTHERS
An ice pack applied to hot, inflamed testicles is very useful in the early stages of orchitis, specially after wounds or other injuries.

REMEDIES: TESTICULAR CANCER

Conventionally, treatment is castration or removal of the affected testicle. Natural medicines can help by the use of remedies for swollen, inflamed testicles (see orchitis) while awaiting neutering, and remedies for treatment of cancer (page 121) while any conventional procedures are being undertaken, and after any conventional treatment, to help prevent spread of the cancer and to prevent recurrence. Check the pet's testicles regularly for lumps or for any change in size or consistency.

ORCHITIS

CAUSES

- injury
- infection

SIGNS AND SYMPTOMS

- painful, swollen testicle
- loss of appetite
- difficulty in passing urine

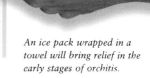

An ice pack wrapped in a towel will bring relief in the early stages of orchitis.

TESTICULAR CANCER

CAUSES

- usually unknown
- failure of testicles to "drop" from abdomen

SIGNS AND SYMPTOMS

- enlargement of a testicle
- changes in sizes of testicles

Penis problems

INJURY

CAUSES

- attack by other pets

SIGNS AND SYMPTOMS

- bleeding
- pain
- visible wound

BALANITIS

CAUSES

- bacterial or viral infection

SIGNS AND SYMPTOMS

- large volume of discharge from sheath
- redness
- pet will lick sheath

PHIMOSIS AND PARAPHIMOSIS

CAUSES

- anatomical defects
- hormonal imbalance

SIGNS AND SYMPTOMS

- **phimosis:** difficulty withdrawing penis back into sheath
- **paraphimosis:** difficulty extruding penis from sheath

There are three main types: injury; difficulty in extracting the penis from or withdrawing it into the sheath; and balanitis.

INJURY

The symptoms of injury are bleeding, pain, and visible wounds. The causes tend to be attacks from other pets – usually in groups of small pets such as gerbils, or when two males are put together in species that normally live alone (such as hamsters).

BALANITIS

Balanitis is excessive discharge from the sheath. Some pets (especially dogs) may produce a fair volume of discharge quite normally. This is usually yellow or green.

The affected pet will lick at sheath, and there is usually visible redness and soreness.

It may follow injury to penis, or be caused by a bacterial infection, occasionally viral infection.

PHIMOSIS AND PARAPHIMOSIS

Phimosis is difficulty in withdrawing the penis back into the sheath. Paraphimosis is difficulty in extruding the penis from the sheath. Both of these conditions are apparent on visual examination.

Penile injury in gerbils is usually the result of an aggressive attack.

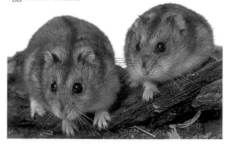

REMEDIES: INJURY

To treat an injured penis, use the same remedies as for wounds (page 179).

REMEDIES: BALANITIS

Conventional treatment prescribes anti-infective agents, but the problem often recurs. Natural medicines offer an effective treatment.

HERBAL
Aloe vera gel, or solution, applied to sheath (externally and inside the sheath) is soothing.

HOMEOPATHY
Calendula lotion applied around sheath.
Acid nit. – where there is ulceration and acute inflammation of the penis or the opening of the sheath.
Hydrastis – when the discharge is thick, stringy, and yellow.
Merc. sol. – for copious, green discharge.
Merc. corr. – thick, green discharge, which may be bloodstained, and causes great irritation and discomfort.
Hepar sulph. – for persistent bacterial infections.
Belladonna – for hot, painful, swollen sheath.
Pulsatilla – for bland, creamy, copious discharge.

REMEDIES: PHIMOSIS AND PARAPHIMOSIS

Treat underlying causes – treat infections or osteodystrophy; surgically correct narrowing of sheath if necessary.

HOMEOPATHY
Picric acid will help diminish prolonged erection of penis in phimosis, with overexcitement, in young dogs.
Yohimbinum will help the penis extruded more from weakness than from overactive hormones.

Hypersexuality and hyposexuality

The hypersexual, or oversexed, male is without doubt a more common problem than the undersexed male in all species (including humans), but natural medicines will help both conditions.

The main symptom is sexual aggression. In most instances of "unsociable" male sexual behavior, the condition causes problems to us, rather than to the pet. Mostly hypersexuality is a problem (for us) in dogs, since in other species the symptoms can be controlled by adjusting housing and environment – in other words, avoiding the males being put in a situation in which their hypersexuality is evident.

In dogs, it is more difficult to control – young male dogs may become aggressive, not only to other dogs, but to people too. They tend to roam, and not come back when called. They mark their territory excessively with urine – and this can extend to areas inside the home. They will mount

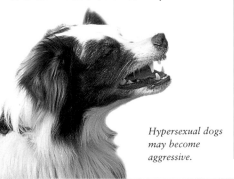

Hypersexual dogs may become aggressive.

REMEDIES: HYPERSEXUALITY

To avoid the necessity for castration, natural medicines can be used.

AROMATHERAPY
Lavender and **sweet marjoram** have a quieting effect on sexual hyperactivity.

HERBAL
Skullcap with **valerian** is calming and soothing, and lowers overactivity of any kind.

FLOWER AND GEM REMEDIES
Vervain – for "over enthusiasm."
Impatiens – for pets that are overexcited but also irritable and snappy.

HOMEOPATHY
Camomile – for young, snappy, irritable, excitable pets.
Picric acid – for prolonged erections and excessive mounting behavior.

---

and be sexually active with cushions, furniture, other animals, and, most embarrassingly, people.

HYPOSEXUALITY

Lack of normal sexual drive is not necessarily a problem, except in animals used for breeding. It is usually caused by hormonal deficiency.

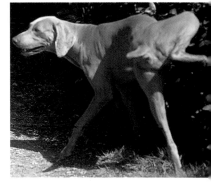

Hypersexual dogs will mark out territory beyond their normal boundaries.

HYPERSEXUALITY

CAUSES

- extension of natural instincts and the naturally occuring male hormone, testosterone

SIGNS AND SYMPTOMS

- sexual aggression
- roaming
- marking territory excessively with urine
- mounting inanimate objects, other animals, and humans

REMEDIES: HYPOSEXUALITY

AROMATHERAPY
Rose, neroli, patchouli, ylang ylang, black pepper, and **sandalwood** all have "aphrodisiac" qualities.

HERBAL
Damiana and **ginseng** can increase a deficient sexual drive.

HOMEOPATHY
Agnus castus – for the older animal in general.
Conium – for lack of erection in older pets.
Lycopodium – for lack of interest in females.
Phos. acid – for young disinterest in females.

Rose has aphrodisiac qualities.

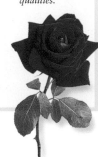

HYPOSEXUALITY

CAUSES

- hormonal deficiency

SIGNS AND SYMPTOMS

- lack of normal sex drive

Immune system disease

The immune system is a complex combination of body processes, which protects the body against infection and disease. These immune processes do not take place in a single organ, and many different protective mechanisms are involved, so it is extremely difficult to identify and discover the reasons for malfunction of the immune system.

It is known that an animal with a weakened immune system is more prone to develop a wide range of infections and other conditions. There is equally no doubt that a pet with a fully functioning immune system is less likely to pick up infections or parasites, is less prone to allergies, and is less likely to develop auto-immune disease.

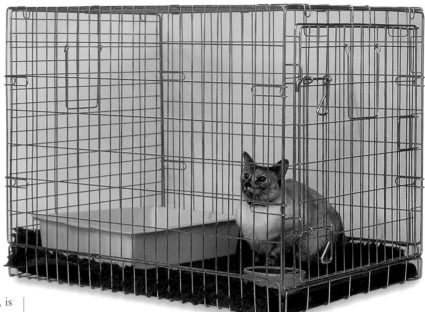

Pets with a weakened immune system are more likely to develop infections.

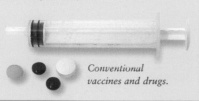

Conventional vaccines and drugs.

There is a controversy about the use of vaccines in pets. Many chronic diseases, such as eczema, colitis, and epilepsy, seem to occur shortly after the use of vaccines. Damage to the immune system could well be triggered by the use of vaccines – particularly the practice of vaccinating pets at a very early age, and then giving them yearly boosters for life. There is no doubt that yearly boosters are not required for all diseases, throughout life. Many veterinarians are now using a more flexible programme of vaccinating every few years, depending on the local incidence of disease, and the health and age of the pet concerned. Always consult your veterinarian if you are worried about the risks of vaccination.

It is not wise to vaccinate pets when they are not fully fit and well, nor is it a good idea to vaccinate them while they are on conventional medication. This could aggravate immune system damage.

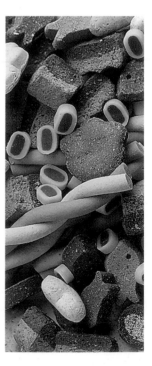

A balanced diet is a significant factor in maintaining a strong immune system.

VACCINES

There are alternatives if vaccination is not appropriate. A combination of natural immune system enhancing remedies, with specific homeopathic remedies that give protection against individual diseases, can be formulated by a veterinarian with expertise in natural medicines.

AUTO-IMMUNE CONDITIONS

Apart from general immune system dysfunction caused by the above factors, a particular set of immune system problems occur, in which the body reacts to its own tissues as if they were foreign and begins to destroy them. These are known as auto-immune conditions and there are several of them.

• Auto-immune hemolytic anemia – the body destroys its own red blood cells (anemia), causing weakness and in some cases jaundice.

• Immune mediated thrombocytopenia – another blood disease, causing persistent hemorrhage. Nose bleeds, blood in feces, and frequent bruising are a feature.

• Systemic lupus erythematosus – this affects many body tissues, especially joints and skin. Lameness, joint swelling, and itchy, red skin are noticeable. A manifestation of this is discoid lupus erythematosus, which affects the skin, nose, face, and ears. There is loss of skin color, loss of fur, and itching. Symptoms are often worse in sunlight.

• Bullous auto-immune skin disease – there are several types of this disease, which is also known as the Pemphigus group of diseases. All cause ulceration and crusting of different areas of the skin.

• Rheumatoid arthritis – causes swollen, painful joints, with stiffness in the mornings.

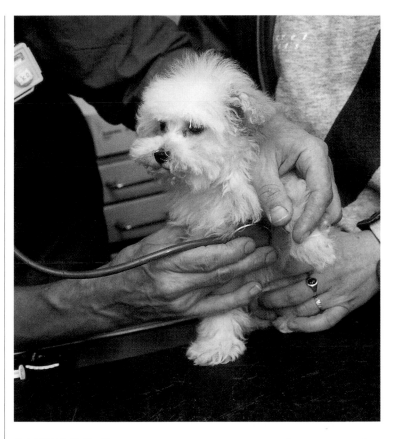

ABOVE There is some controversy over the routine use of vaccines in pets.

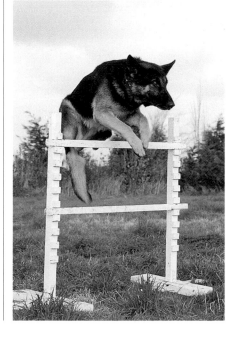

LEFT Immune dysfunction can lead to the loss of healthy joints and normal activity.

Other auto-immune diseases

Many conditions are now being discovered to be caused by auto-immune disease. These include CDRM in dogs (see page 120), hypothyroidism (see page 102) and keratoconjunctivitis sicca (dry eye, see page 85). There may be other conditions which result from immune disease that as yet have not been recognized.

Auto-immune disease in most cases appears to be caused by a genetic defect. However, it also seems that in individuals with a genetic susceptibility to developing auto-immune disease, there are "trigger factors" that make the dormant" disease active. These trigger factors are those described at the start of this section – nutritional, environmental, stress, and the administration of drugs and vaccines.

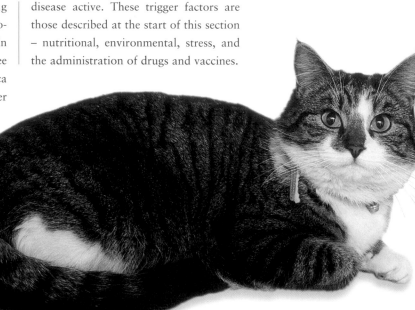

REMEDIES

AROMATHERAPY

Tea tree – antiviral, antibacterial, and antifungal, and has a stimulating action on the entire immune system. It is ideal to use where infections have entered the body because the immune system is damaged. It is able to kill many bacteria that are now immune to antibiotics.
Bergamot – stimulates the production of white blood cells (one of the immune system's many defenses), and has a general uplifting effect, helping to combat stress.

Geranium relieves stress and balances the hormonal system.

Eucalyptus and **thyme** – both have antiviral properties, as well as boosting the immune system's general defense against infection.
Lavender – strengthens the whole immune system, increases white blood cell production, and helps remove toxins from the body, so reducing the likelihood of pollutants and drugs damaging the immune system.
Geranium – a stress-relieving, uplifting remedy, and also balances the hormonal system, which is closely linked with the immune system.
Ylang ylang – a calming, antistress remedy, which also ensures deep, restful sleep, enabling healing and repair of damaged tissues to take place more rapidly.

HERBAL

Echinacea – an ideal immune system booster, cleanses and purifies the blood and lymphatic system, stimulates the production of white blood cells and antibodies, and is particularly effective at dealing with infections entering damaged skin.

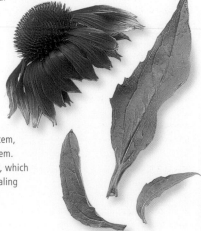

Echinacea is a powerful system cleanser and tonic.

Natural remedies can boost the immune system and help ensure the well-being of your pet.

TREATING AUTO-IMMUNE DISEASE

Any condition in which immune system weakness is a factor, involves:

• Removing as many of the trigger factors as possible. Pay attention to diet and look at stress levels to ensure environment is as ideal as possible.

• Restrict the use of conventional drugs and vaccines. This will need discussion with your own veterinary practice and their liaison with any veterinarian specializing in natural therapies to whom you may have been referred, or are obtaining advice.

• Treating any symptoms the immune condition is causing – see the medicines suggested in this book for any specific symptoms your pet may have.

• Giving specific immune system boosters (see below).

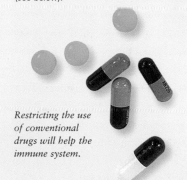

Restricting the use of conventional drugs will help the immune system.

Garlic – enhances the ability of the immune system to resist infection at all levels, especially in the respiratory system. Like tea tree essential oil, it can eliminate some infections that are now immune to antibiotics.

Ginseng – improves circulation, promotes white blood cell production, eases stress symptoms, and helps the body cope with toxins.

Licorice – another herb with stress-relieving properties, and an ability to promote production of white blood cells and antibodies.

HOMEOPATHY
It is not the remedy that cures the condition, but the remedy "encouraging" or "reminding" the body how to heal itself. For immune system disease, treat the symptoms with the appropriate homeopathic remedies, but most importantly, see a homeopathic veterinarian who has expertise enough to prescribe the correct constitutional remedy.

This will be deep-acting and provide an effective immune system booster.

FLOWER AND GEM REMEDIES
Amaranthus – for weakened, debilitated animals with immune system damage.
Pansy – an antiviral agent in particular.
McCartney rose – especially for leukemia, and general immune system problems.

NUTRITIONAL
The anti-oxidant **vitamins, A, C,** and **E,** combine well to boost the immune system.
B-complex (especially B6) – is also beneficial.
Zinc – strengthens the immune system.
Proantho cyanidins – anti-allergic and help treat cancers that develop as a result of immune system disorder.
Other supplements include **chlorella, royal jelly,** and **kelp** – see pages 14-15 on Supplements and the Immune System.

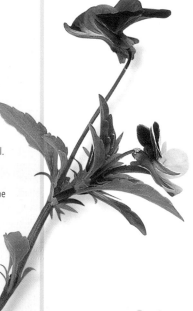

Pansy is useful as an antiviral agent and boosts the immune system.

Lymph disorders

CAUSES

- infection
- cancer

SIGNS AND SYMPTOMS

- visibly enlarged lymph gland(s)
- general malaise

The lymphatic system is the immune system's "drainage channel;" the lymph glands are "detoxifying" points along the route. Although linked with the circulation in general, the lymphatic system has its own set of diseases.

Apart from pressure at any point in the lymphatic system causing fluid build-up (treat the cause of the problem, and also treat as for edema, see page 98), the main problem affecting the lymph system is enlarged lymph glands. For treatment of cancerous lymph glands, see section on cancer (page 121). Symptoms of lymph gland enlargements are:

- One or more palpably or visibly enlarged lymph glands, general malaise.

Causes include:

- Lymphosarcoma – this is a cancer of the lymph glands. Occurs in dogs, possibly from a viral cause, and in cats, caused by feline leukemia virus. Often noticeable first in dogs when the lymph glands of the neck become swollen.
- Lymphadenopathy – non-cancerous swelling of lymph glands. May affect a single gland – or all lymph glands. Usually caused by the lymph glands reacting to infection.

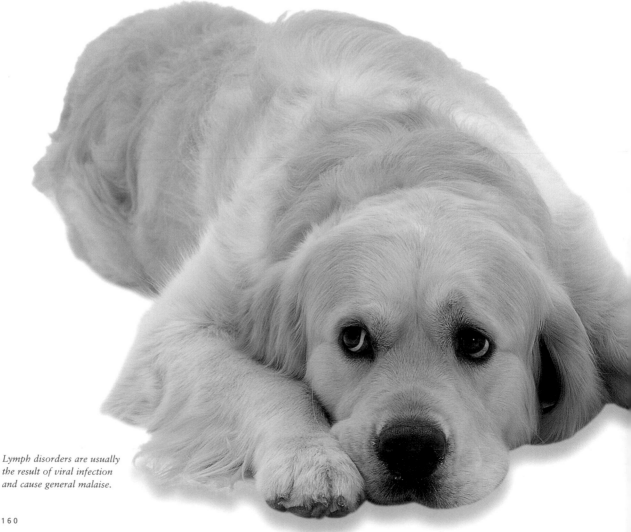

Lymph disorders are usually the result of viral infection and cause general malaise.

REMEDIES

Guinea pigs are prone to a form of lympha-denopathy called "cervical lymphadenitis," or simply "lumps." As with all lymph disorders, treat it naturally as follows:

AROMATHERAPY

Celery seed is a depurative – that is, it combats impurities in blood, lymph, and other organs. As such, it is a useful treatment for lymphadenitis.
Coriander/Cilantro – another depurative essential oil, and also antibacterial, so ideal for infection in lymph glands.

CRYSTAL AND GEM ESSENCES

Jet and **ruby** are both used as treatments for glandular swellings of all kinds, from all causes.

HOMEOPATHY

Belladonna – for hot, swollen lymph glands, tender to the touch. The affected pet may be feverish and thirsty.
Bryonia – for hard, swollen lymph glands. The patient will feel better for the glands being firmly pressed, and is also better when resting and worse when moving.

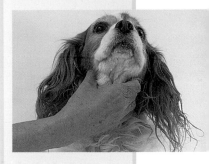

Guinea pigs can suffer from an infection causing swelling of one or all lymph glands.

Bufo. – for abscesses in lymph glands, and for hard nodules of lymph tissue in mammary glands.
Calc. carb. – for enlarged lymph nodes in heavily built pets, who tend to be inactive, overweight, and need warmth and plenty of food.
Baryta carb. – for multiple lymph gland enlargement in very young pets, or in the elderly animal. Baryta carb. always helps problems of the very young, or very old.
Calc. fluor – for very hard "stony" enlargements of lymph glands, often enlarging very slowly.
Conium – for hardened, enlarged lymph glands in elderly animals, often with noticeable hind-quarter weakness.
Camomile – enlarged lymph glands in young pets, often associated with teething pains, sore gums, and sore eyes and ears.
Phytolacca – a classic homeopathic remedy for lymph gland disease. Swollen glands, often firm, red, and sensitive. Especially good for tender throat lymph glands, and for sore throats in general. Helps treat cancerous lymph glands.

HERBAL

Echinacea – an immune system booster, and particularly good at stimulating healing of lymph gland infections.

NUTRITIONAL

Apple cider vinegar applied to swollen glands is soothing and healing. **Vitamins C** and **B-complex** promote healing in lymph gland disease.

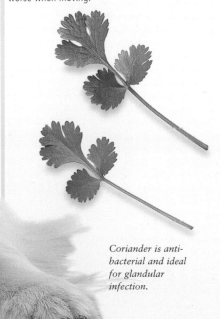

Coriander is anti-bacterial and ideal for glandular infection.

DOS AND DON'TS

Don't assume lumps that appear are cysts or warts. They may be skin tumors or enlarged lymph glands. All swellings that appear and grow quickly should be examined by a veterinarian.

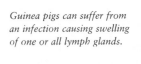

A veterinarian should examine any lumps or swellings that have suddenly developed, or grown rapidly.

Do remember that enlarged lymph glands may cause difficulty in swallowing – give soft, easily swallowed food – and breathing – avoid stress and excitement.

Parasites

CAUSES

- transmission from other hosts

SIGNS AND SYMPTOMS

- visible evidence of parasites
- excessive scratching or grooming
- raised red bumps on the skin

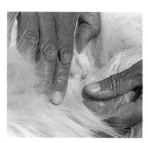

ABOVE *Ticks are usually picked up from long grass. They attach themselves via their mouth parts and do not move.*

RIGHT *In its life cycle, the flea feeds from a host, and lays eggs, which hatch and the new fleas then find themselves other hosts, and the cycle continues.*

Parasites are creatures that live on or in another animal and feed on it in some way. A healthy lifestyle and a balanced, natural diet should help to ensure that parasites are kept to a minimum, but even the healthiest, fittest pet will occasionally be host to internal parasites such as worms, and to external (surface-dwelling) parasites.

Natural medicines can play an important role both in preventing parasites, and in resolving any infestation that does occur. Although most pets can potentially be affected by a wide range of parasites, there are certain parasites that are more likely to be found in each individual species:

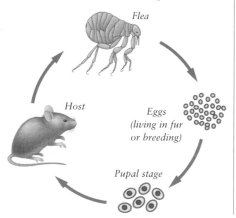

Flea

Host

Eggs
(living in fur
or breeding)

Pupal stage

PARASITES

- **Chinchillas,** are more often affected by ringworm and intestinal worms.
- **Gerbils,** by ringworm, mange mites, and intestinal worms.
- **Hamsters,** by ringworm and mange mites.
- **Rabbits,** by ringworm, ear mites, and mange mites.
- **Rats and mice,** by ringworm and intestinal worms.
- **Ferrets,** by fleas, mange mites, surface mites, ear mites, and ringworm.
- **Birds,** by lice, intestinal worms, and feather mites.
- **Tortoises and terrapins,** by intestinal worms.
- **Cats,** by intestinal worms, fleas, ticks, ear mites, and surface mites.
- **Dogs,** by fleas, lice, ticks, ear mites, mange mites, surface mites, and intestinal worms (full house as far as dogs are concerned!).
- **Fish,** by intestinal worms, fungi (treat as for ringworm), crustaceans, flukes, and protozoa (treat as for fleas, lice, and ticks).

FLEAS, LICE, AND TICKS

These are all surface-dwelling parasites. Fleas are small, dark brown insects that run rapidly through the fur; lice are tiny, gray insects that move very slowly and form clusters, particularly on the ear flaps; ticks resemble smooth, gray warts. They fix their mouth parts into the skin and do not move.

Symptoms to look out for are the visible evidence of parasites – an affected pet may scratch and groom excessively and, if the patient is hypersensitive to flea bites (i.e. allergic to flea saliva), there may be raised, red bumps on the skin.

REMEDIES

AROMATHERAPY
Cedarwood, eucalyptus, terebinth, lemon, rosemary, and **lavender** all help to prevent external parasites. They can be given by massage or added to water (three drops per ⅔ cup/150 ml water) and combed or brushed into fur.

HOMEOPATHY
Sulfur – one dose should be given weekly to prevent flea infestations.
Pulex – is a soothing treatment for flea irritation.

HERBAL
Pennyroyal, tansy, and **fleabane** are flea-repelling herbs.
Garlic is also very effective: one third of a chopped clove should be added to food daily.

NUTRITIONAL
Brewer's yeast may be given by mouth, or brushed into the fur.
Cider vinegar – at a rate of 1 teaspoon per 2½ cups of drinking water – is another good preventive measure. Bathing in dilute vinegar helps eliminate fleas.

MITES

Mites are tiny parasites, too small to be seen with the naked eye. There are three main groups of mites: surface, mange, and ear mites.

SURFACE MITES

Surface mites live on the surface of the skin and cause irritation leading to scratching and itching. Two common species are cheyletiella – the rabbit fur mite (found on several species, not just on rabbits) – and harvest mites – orange mites affecting feet, legs, and stomach, mainly in the fall. Treat surface mites as for fleas, lice and ticks (see pages 162 and 165). Feather mites in birds are surface mites.

MANGE MITES

Mange mites are burrowing mites, living deep inside the skin and causing intense irritation, often with secondary infection of the skin. The two commonest types of mange mites are sarcoptic demodectic mange. The first is especially common in dogs, often picked up from foxes, and potentially transmissible to humans (known as scabies when affecting people). The second usually occurs when the immune system is damaged. Treat with immune system boosters as well as the remedies below.

EAR MITES

Ear mites live inside ears, where they cause intense irritation, a large amount of discharge (usually dry, crumbly, and black in dogs, cats, and ferrets, and yellowish-white in rabbits), and visible head–shaking or ear–scratching. Ear mites are a common cause of aural hematoma (see page 78) and are most common in young animals, especially kittens.

REMEDIES

AROMATHERAPY
Lemongrass, lavender, lemon, and **rosemary** may be used by massage, or diluted (3 drops per ⅔ cup) 150 ml of water and brushed into the fur daily to treat mites. **Basil, citronella, Virginia cedarwood,** and **cinammon leaf** can be used in a similar way as mite "repellents" to help protect pets against mites.

FLOWER AND GEM REMEDIES
Cotton – effective against mange mites.

HOMEOPATHY
Sulfur – especially if patient prefers not to be too hot.
Psorinum – especially for pets who love the heat.
Bovista – where face is particularly affected with intense itching.

HERBAL
Garlic is a good remedy for all parasite problems.

Lemongrass can be brushed into fur to treat mites.

- surface mites: scratching and itching
- mange mites: intense irritation, often with secondary skin infection
- ear mites: itense, large amount of discharge, head–shaking or ear–scratching

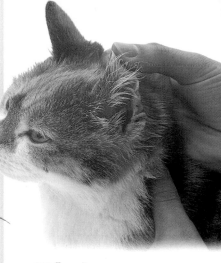

ABOVE *Ear mites are a common problem, especially in young cats.*

REMEDIES

Treat them in the folllowing ways:

HOMEOPATHY
Sulfur – for patients that avoid heat and prefer to be cool.
Psorinum – for pets that love warmth.
Rhus tox. – for severe itching and soreness of ears.
Graphites – if discharge is thick, sticky, and smelly.

HERBAL
A mixture of equal parts of **thyme, rosemary,** and **rue** infusions, mixed 50:50 with olive oil is an effective ear-cleansing remedy, which will kill mites at the same time.
Olive oil and **vitamin E** (3 teaspoons of olive oil with 500 iu vitamin E) will clean and heal the damaged, inflamed ear canal.

Ringworm

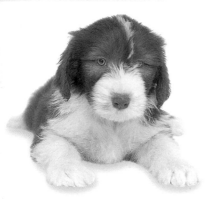

ABOVE *Young pets are susceptible to ringworm and other parasites.*

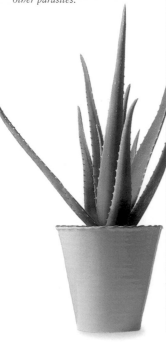

This is a fungal skin parasite that is transmitted between most species of pets and is transmissible to humans. Although pets are often blamed for passing on ringworm to children, the most common source of ringworm in these cases is, in fact, other children.

The symptoms are usually, but not always, circular particles of hair loss, with the affected areas of skin red and sore.

REMEDIES

There are several species of fungus causing ringworm. Some, but not all, exhibit the strange phenomenon of glowing under ultraviolet light – a greenish fluorescence. Treat with the following:

AROMATHERAPY

Geranium, patchouli, lavender, myrrh, tea tree, and **tagetes** are all effective remedies. They can be administered by massage or diluted (three drops in ⅔ cup/150 ml water) and brushed into the fur.

HOMEOPATHY

Bacillinum – a classic homeopathic remedy for ringworm.
   Sepia – small, circular, itchy spots.
   Tellurium – circular lesions, distributed evenly on both sides of the body.
      Kali. arsen. – dry, scaly patches with severe itching.

HERBAL

Apply **echinacea** or **goldenseal** tincture to affected area daily.
Aloe vera gel is soothing and cooling for inflamed areas of skin.

Aloe vera gel can be used to soothe and cool skin irritated by ringworm.

INTESTINAL WORMS

Roundworms and tapeworms in the intestinal tract are all too common, especially in young pets. Tapeworms are carried by fleas, so flea-infested pets are most at risk. Other worms found in pets include hookworms, whipworms, lungworms, and heartworms, but these are much less common.

Symptoms to look out for are worms that may be visible in the feces. Roundworms are thin, white, round-bodied, and up to 6 in (15 cm) long; tapeworms appear as flat, short segments (the main tapeworm remains in the intestine). Each tapeworm segment that is passed can move, and is full of eggs.

TAPEWORM CYCLE

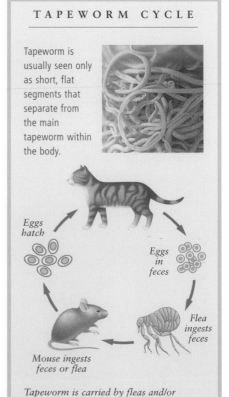

Tapeworm is usually seen only as short, flat segments that separate from the main tapeworm within the body.

Eggs hatch

Eggs in feces

Flea ingests feces

Mouse ingests feces or flea

Tapeworm is carried by fleas and/or small animals, and then ingested by pet.

ROUNDWORM CYCLE

Roundworms are a common parasite. They are thin, white worms that can grow to be 6in (15cm) long

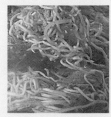

Ingestion by bitches of expelled eggs in puppies feces

Bitch infects puppies via suckling or uterus

Puppy

Eggs in feces

Roundworms are ingested as eggs and develop in the body of the pet.

CAUSES

- transmission via fleas or mice (tapeworm)
- swallowing eggs passed by other animals (roundworm)

SIGNS AND SYMPTOMS

- worms visible in feces

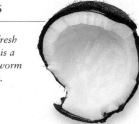

RIGHT *Fleas leave feces, which look like specks of grit*

BELOW *Grooming your pet with a flea comb to eliminate fleas will also reduce the incidence of tapeworms.*

REMEDIES

Treat intestinal worms with:

AROMATHERAPY
Bergamot, thyme, and **marjoram** may all be used for massage when a pet has an infestation of worms.

HOMEOPATHY
Cina and **Chenopodium** are effective for helping to eliminate roundworms; **Granatum** or **Filix mas.** is suitable for an infestation of tapeworms. In each case, give one dose twice daily for three days, every four weeks, as a preventive measure.

Grated fresh coconut is a natural worm repellent.

NUTRITIONAL
Chopped papaya and **grated coconut, melon pips, grated carrot, ground pumpkin seeds,** and **pomegranate** oil are all worm-repellent. Give a mixture of some or all of these regularly – up to 1 teaspoon daily.

FLEA AND WORM TREATMENT

Most veterinarians suggest routinely and regularly giving flea and worm treatments to prevent pets being infested with parasites. It is wise to dose young pets – especially puppies and kittens – for worms, as they always have intestinal

worms. Adult pets, if healthy, are unlikely to be affected by an appreciable number of worms, and do not necessarily need frequent dosing.

Long-term treatment for fleas is questionable, as many flea preparations are potentially damaging to the pet, to us, and to the environment. It is preferable to treat major flea infestations with conventional insecticides, but use natural methods at other times.

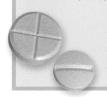

Worm treatments should be given to young pets.

Specific infectious diseases

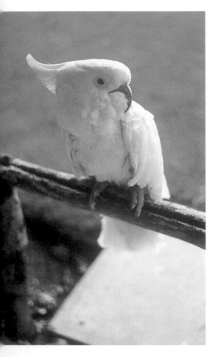

Cockatoos and other caged birds are prone to psittacosis, which causes weakness, diarrhea, and weight loss.

Each species of pet has its own specific infectious diseases, caused by viruses, bacteria, fungi, and other organisms. For reasons of space, only the most important infections in each species are included here.

BIRDS

Mycoplasma – a respiratory infection, with discharge from nostrils, depression, weakness.

Psittacosis (also known as ornithosis): diarrhea, weakness, weight loss, eye discharge.

CATS

Feline leukemia virus – this affects the immune system, causing a range of symptoms, including anemia and kidney and liver damage.

Feline infectious enteritis – a viral infection that results in acute fever, vomiting, and severe diarrhea; these symptoms will lead to rapid dehydration and often death.

Cats are subject to several serious feline viral infections with a variety of symptoms.

Feline immunodeficiency virus – related to HIV, the human virus linked to AIDS. The virus damages a cat's immune system and causes a wide range of symptoms.

Feline infectious anemia – caused by a parasite called hemobartonella, which destroys red blood cells. This causes anemia and weakness.

Feline upper respiratory tract disease (cat flu) – this is caused by two viruses. Feline viral rhinotracheitis causes coughing, sneezing, and nasal discharge. It can be fatal. Surviving cats often have persistent "snuffles." Feline calicivirus causes milder flu symptoms, often with mouth ulcers.

Feline infectious peritonitis – a viral infection that can cause two sets of symptoms. The "wet" form results in a build-up of fluid in the abdomen, with weight loss and weakness: the "dry" form causes weakness and weight loss, but no fluid build-up. In both cases, the symptoms may worsen and lead to jaundice (most obvious as a "yellowing" of the whites of the eyes), vomiting, diarrhea, and consequently dehydration.

Toxoplasmosis – this protozoal infection affects various parts of the body. The many symptoms include weight loss, nasal discharge, coughing, diarrhea, and abortion. Toxoplasmosis can be transmitted to humans, so great care should be taken by pregnant women when handling cats.

Chlamydia – this is an organism that causes conjunctivitis, eye discharge, and sometimes sneezing and nasal discharge. It can cause infertility or abortion.

CHINCHILLAS

Listeriois – causes depression, diarrhea, loss of appetite. White nodules in liver found after death.

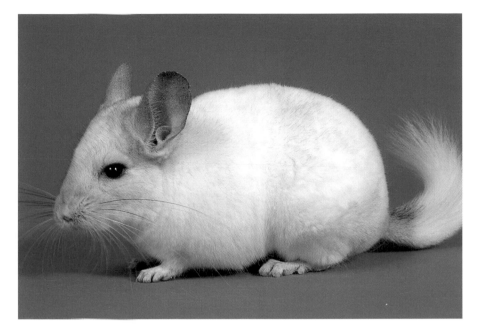

Chinchillas can be affected by several specific infections with common symptoms such as diarrhea.

DOGS

Canine parvovirus – a viral infection, this disease affects both the digestive system and the heart, causing severe vomiting and diarrhea with blood. In young puppies, it may also result in heart damage.

Distemper – a viral infection that affects many parts of the body. The symptoms include fever, coughing, nasal discharge, conjunctivitis, diarrhea, and convulsions (fits) or chorea.

Canine hepatitis – this viral infection attacks a dog's liver, causing vomiting, diarrhea, fever, abdominal pain, and in some rare cases jaundice.

Canine leptospirosis – there are two forms of this bacterial infection. One form affects the liver and causes jaundice, diarrhea, and vomiting; the other causes kidney damage, and produces accompanying symptoms of mouth ulcers, excessive thirst, and vomiting.

Kennel cough – a combination of viral and bacterial infection, kennel cough is prevalent in situations where there are many dogs, such as at boarding kennels or dog shows, enabling the rapid transmission of the disease. It affects the respiratory system, resulting in a sore throat and persistent coughing.

Lyme disease – this is a bacterial disease spread by ticks. This mainly affects the musculoskeletal system, resulting in obvious lameness, but it can also cause heart damage.

Aspergillosis – this is a fungal infection affecting the respiratory system. It causes nasal discharge, coughing, and sometimes epistaxis (nose bleeds).

Neosporosis – this is a protozoal disease that affects the musculoskeletal system, causing paralysis and stiffness of the legs (usually the hind legs).

Tetanus – a bacterial infection that affects the nervous system. It causes muscle stiffness and paralysis, especially of the jaw.

Toxoplasmosis – another protozoal infection. It affects various parts of the body and produces a number of different symptoms, including weight loss, coughing, nasal discharge, diarrhea, and abortions in bitches.

Dogs are vulnerable to a number of specific infectious diseases. Some, like kennel cough, can be contagious.

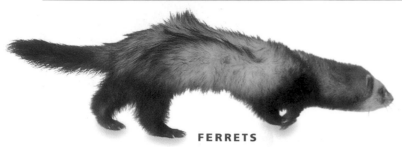

Ferrets can be infected with canine distemper.

FERRETS

Canine distemper – ferrets are susceptible to distemper. Fever, discharge from eyes and nose. Rash under chin and in groin. Later, convulsions occur. Transmitted from dogs.

Human influenza virus – listlessness, high temperature, nasal discharge.

Aleutian disease – a virus infection. Black, tarry feces, recurrent fever, weight loss, aggression, hypersensitivity, thyroid inflammation, paralysis of hindquarters.

GERBILS

Tyzzer's disease – symptoms include lethargy, loss of weight, loss of appetite.

Salmonellosis – look out for diarrhea, staring (out of condition) coat, dehydration.

GUINEA PIGS

Streptococcal pneumonia – gasping, nasal discharge; is rapidly fatal.

Cervical lymphadenitis – infected purulent lymph nodes of the neck, caused by streptococcus.

Pseudotuberculosis – diarrhea, weight loss, enlarged lymph nodes. Animal usually dies within 3–4 weeks.

HAMSTERS

Tyzzer's disease – acute diarrhoea, rapidly leading to death.

Bacterial pneumonia – nasal discharge, difficulty in breathing. Usually triggered by stress.

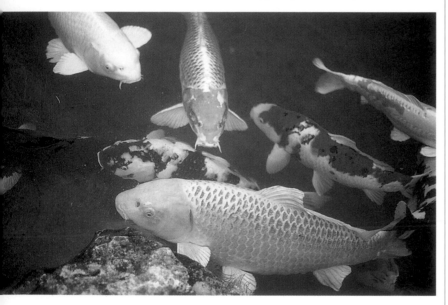

Most specific infections in fish are evident from abnormalities in the skin.

FISH

Spring viremia of carp – caught from imported fish; symptoms are sick fish, weak and dark color, and hanging in the water.

Fish tuberculosis – lumpy swellings on the skin as well as internal lumps. Transmissible to humans (known as "aquarist's arm").

Ulcer disease of goldfish – bacterial infection causing ulcers and furrows in the skin of the affected fish.

White spot (Ich.) – white spots on skin; a protozoal disease.

Saproleynia – a fungal infection looking like white "tufts" growing on the skin.

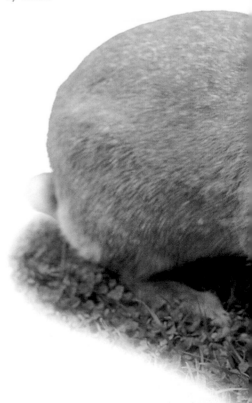

RABBITS

Clostridial enterotoxemia – rapid onset bowel infection, diarrhea; animal often dies within 24 hours.

Tyzzer's disease – diarrhea, loss of weight. Diarrhea often bloodstained.

Pasteurellosis – most frequent single cause of illness in rabbits. Purulent discharge from nose and eyes. May spread to middle ear or lungs.

Myxomatosis – spread via the rabbit flea from wild rabbits. Swelling of eyelids with purulent conjunctivitis; later, swelling of head and neck. Almost always fatal.

RATS AND MICE

Tyzzer's disease – diarrhea, weight loss, weakness.

Salmonellosis – diarrhea, loss of condition, often fatal.

SNAKES AND LIZARDS

Viral respiratory disease – gasping, blowing bubbles, lethargy.

TORTOISES AND TERRAPINS

Flagellate infection – increased thirst, poor appetite, diarrhea.

Viral rhinitis – continuous thin, watery nasal discharge, breathing through an open mouth, noisy breathing. Sometimes conjunctivitis and watery discharge from eyes.

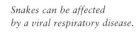

Snakes can be affected by a viral respiratory disease.

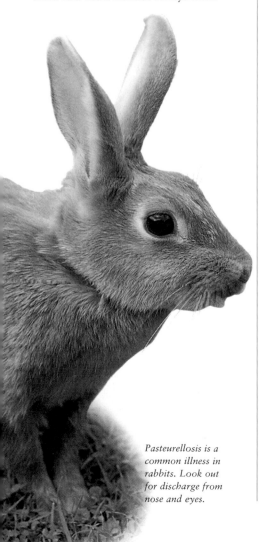

Pasteurellosis is a common illness in rabbits. Look out for discharge from nose and eyes.

REMEDIES

Specific infections should always be treated with natural remedies that correspond to the particular symptoms of the infection.

Apart from choosing natural medicines that are appropriate for the individual nature of the disease, there are some general anti-infective remedies available, which are shown below. In acute bacterial infections, antibiotics are necessary, and can be life-saving. However, long courses of antibiotics should be avoided whenever possible. After a course of antibiotics, always give a course of probiotics, to restore the population of "beneficial" gut bacteria to normal.

AROMATHERAPY
Atlas cedarwood is antifungal.
Rosewood is generally anti-infective, especially for sudden onset of infection.
Camphor is generally anti-infective.

Lemongrass treats most infectious diseases.
Lemon eucalyptus is antifungal and antiviral.
Lavender is antifungal.
Tea tree is antibacterial, antiviral, and antifungal.
Nutmeg is antibacterial.
Geranium is antifungal.
Black pepper is antiviral.
Patchouli is antifungal.

FLOWER AND GEM REMEDIES
Pansy is antiviral.

NUTRITIONAL
Vitamin C is generally anti-infective.
Radishes are antibacterial and antifungal.

Nutmeg is a natural antibacterial remedy.

Mental and behavioral problems

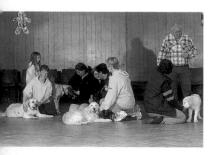

As well as obedience training, dog training classes provide extended socialization.

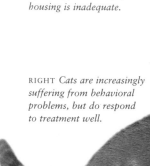

ABOVE *Caged birds show signs of stress, particularly if their housing is inadequate.*

RIGHT *Cats are increasingly suffering from behavioral problems, but do respond to treatment well.*

Behavioral problems in dogs seem to be on the increase and many dogs exhibit the same kinds of anxieties or hyperactivity seen in some children and adults. To help prevent the development of such problems, the factors discussed here should be borne in mind.

If behavior problems have developed, seek advice quickly. Trained behavior counselors can solve many problems.

MAJOR FACTORS

- Only go to see a litter whose parents you know to be calm and well-behaved. Choose a puppy that is neither shy and withdrawn when handled, nor too bouncy and boisterous.
- One common reason for problems of fear and aggression in young dogs is lack of proper socialization: between 6 and 12 weeks of age, puppies must be introduced to dogs and humans of all shapes and sizes, and learn how to react normally to them without fear and apprehension.
- Train your puppy – dog-training classes are helpful, but training must also be carried through to everyday activities. Do not let your puppy become dominant in the home by allowing him or her to sleep in your bed, to sit on chairs, to eat before you do, or to pull on the lead while out on walks.
- A good, well-balanced diet produces a good, well-balanced dog. Vitamin deficiencies, protein excess, and mineral imbalance can all lead to or aggravate behavioral problems.

When additional help is needed, natural medicines can come into their own.

Cats also seem to be suffering more from behavior problems – aggression, anxiety, inappropriate toileting in the home. Behavior therapy is equally applicable to cats, but again, natural medicines are very effective, either on their own or as a back-up to behavior therapy.

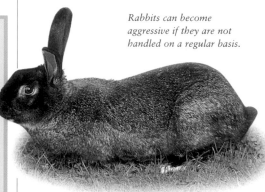

Rabbits can become aggressive if they are not handled on a regular basis.

SMALL PETS

- Small pets show fewer examples of behavior problems.
- Rabbits can become aggressive, especially if receiving little human contact.
- Overcrowding, inappropriate housing, and insufficient space and exercise are the commonest reasons for small pets to show behavior problems.

NERVOUSNESS AND ANXIETY

Accidents, physical or mental abuse by humans, or even undergoing a routine vaccination can lead to anxiety. Some pets are frightened of thunderstorms; some are scared of other pets or vacuum cleaners. Such anxieties can affect pets at different levels. Be sure to choose your pet carefully, with particular consideration to temperament, not just looks.

REMEDIES

Treat nervousness and anxiety with:

AROMATHERAPY
Massage with **camomile, lavender, lemon balm, neroli,** or **sweet marjoram** will have a calming effect.

HOMEOPATHY
Aconite – for nervousness that begins after a frightening experience.
Argent. nit. – for the "hurried and worried" pet.
Gelsemium – for a pet that becomes almost rigid with fear.
Phosphorus – especially for fear of sudden or very loud noises.
Arsen. alb. – for restlessness and anticipatory anxiety (worried about impending event).
Borax – for fear of sudden noises, especially gunshot. Also, often a fear of downward movement.
Ignatia – for pets that become anxious when left on their own.

HERBAL
Camomile is soothing, as is **common oat.**
Hops given as a herbal infusion are extremely helpful for a neurotic pet.
Passiflora will pacify and soothe an anxious pet.
Vervain infusion is another good choice for lack of confidence.
Skullcap with **valerian** – available as proprietary tablets – makes a classic herbal calming remedy.

FLOWER AND GEM REMEDIES
Aspen for general fears and anxieties. Apprehensive when meeting a stranger.
Cerato – pets that lack confidence, needing reassurance from their owners.
Honeysuckle – anxiety in a new home, or while in boarding kennels; homesickness.
Larch – nervousness on meeting people. Pets hide behind you, or disappear into their cage.
Mimulus – for a fear of something specific, such as thunder, fireworks, other animals; any major phobia.
Red chestnut – anxious when others (pets or people) are ill or upset.
Rock rose – for panic and terror after an accident or shock, or being attacked by another animal.

CRYSTAL AND GEM ESSENCES
Aquamarine – a calming, soothing stone, which alleviates fears and phobias.
Peach aventurina – heals emotional traumas and relieves anxiety and fears.
Blue calcite – calming and quieting for nervous pets.
Chrysocholla – calms and soothes fractious animals.
Kyanite – restores confidence of pets that are nervous and do not settle in after homing from rescue centers.
Lepidolite – for anxiety and nervousness in general, also to help break pets of bad habits.
Peridot – a stress-relieving remedy for stressed, anxious pets.
Tourmaline – for fears and phobias, especially fear of thunder and fireworks.
Tourmaline quartz – for pets that become anxious when unwell physically.

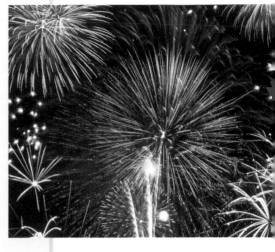

Fireworks and thunder storms can cause many pets to feel nervous or distressed.

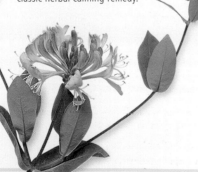

Honeysuckle as a flower remedy is effective in alleviating anxiety and homesickness.

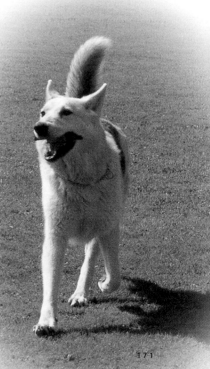

Do not let your dog be dominant or roam freely when out walking in public.

Aggression

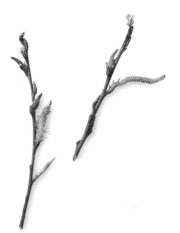

Some species such as this Siamese Fighting Fish have a natural inclination to show aggression.

Pets may become aggressive to other animals of their own species, to other people, or even to their owners. In small pets this is usually a result of over-crowding or insufficient handling. In cats and dogs, most aggression to people is due to poor socialization in the young kitten or puppy, and insufficient training in the growing dog. Cocker spaniels are prone to a severe form of aggression known as Cocker rage syndrome – episodes of serious aggression occur for no known reason.

ABOVE Willow is helpful when pets feel resentment toward a newcomer in the family.

REMEDIES

Behavior therapy will always be helpful treatment and may be essential in severe cases.

AROMATHERAPY
Many essential oils are calming and soothing. Chief of these are:

Angelica root   **Neroli**
Benzoin   **Clary sage**
Cypress   **Vetivert**

All these oils are helpful in promoting a restful, calm atmosphere, in which aggression is much less likely to occur.

HERBAL
Camomile – for irritable, snappy pets. Especially young animals, and particularly when teething.
Gentian – for hysterical and aggressive pets.
Hops – a calming, quieting remedy.
Skullcap and **valerian** – this combination is a classic remedy to remove fears and phobias, and aggressive instincts. It calms and quiets, without making pets sedated or confused, as conventional tranquilizers often do.

FLOWER AND GEM REMEDIES
Beech – for pets that over-react to little things, such as flying off the handle if their bed is moved. They like things their own way and let you know it.
Cherry plum – for pets that snap or bite from fear or stress but are sorry afterward.
Chicory – for pets that like to rule the roost and tell other pets (or people) what to do. They can become snappy if not given their own way.
Holly – for feelings of anger, hatred, envy, and jealousy; often attack new pets (or people) introduced into the home.

Vine – for dominant animals that become aggressive if their dominance is threatened.
Willow – for resentment and bitter feelings, perhaps to a newcomer in the family, or after an operation, or after being attacked.
Tiger lily – for aggression, biting, scratching, hostility of any kind.

HOMEOPATHY
Belladonna – angry animals with a tendency to bite and strike. May have dilated pupils when angry, and be very sensitive to touch.
Hyosycamus – rage beyond any reason; good for Cocker rage syndrome.
Camomile – snappishness and aggression, especially in young, teething animals.
Lachesis – aggression because of jealousy, a newcomer to the house, or other disruption to routine that makes the pet feel less attention is being lavished on them.
Nux vomica – irritable, especially in noisy surroundings. May snap because of this irritability.
Sepia – moody and bad-tempered females, often with hormone imbalance.
Staphisagria – resentment after an operation, a move of home, or the introduction of a new pet.

CRYSTAL AND GEM ESSENCES
Celestite – calms snappy, aggressive pets.
Rhodochrosite – for resentment and irritation.
Rose quartz – for aggressive, over-dominant pets.

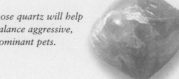

Rose quartz will help balance aggressive, dominant pets.

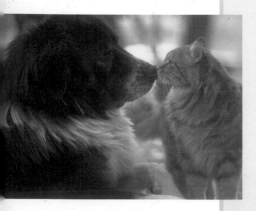

ABOVE Aggression between species is usually the result of poor socialization.

Hyperactivity

A distinction needs to be drawn between normal, enthusiastic high spirits and true hyperactivity, in which persistent wakefulness, repetitive behavior, and manic activity are evident. Stress is probably the most common cause. Hyperactivity can also sometimes be linked to food additives, in which case foods with colorings, flavorings, and other additives should be avoided. There is also some evidence that high levels of protein in the diet of dogs can predispose to hyperactivity, so this should be avoided by ensuring a balanced diet.

Probably the main reason for hyperactivity is the genetic make-up of the pet concerned. Some breeds of dogs – especially Boxers, Border Collies, and Dalmatians – seem more likely to become hyperactive. Environment, however, does play a major part. A noisy atmosphere is more likely to encourage hyperactivity.

Normal play should not be confused with hyperactivity.

REMEDIES

Natural remedies are very effective in treating hyperactivity. Conventional medicine relies on sedatives and tranquilizers or neutering.

AROMATHERAPY
Lavender – a good remedy for nervous tension, stress, and overactivity.
Camomile (German) – for nervous stress, insomnia, good for colds and fevers that may aggravate hyperactivity.
Sweet marjoram – for insomnia, nervous tension, and stress.
Yarrow – calming and soothing for the nervous system, good for high blood pressure and insomnia.
Ylang ylang – an effective "balancer" for depression and for nervous tension, insomnia.

FLOWER AND GEM REMEDIES
Vervain has a soothing effect on a hyperactive pet that tends to become obsessive, and is impulsive, is often tense, and doesn't want to go to bed at night.
White chestnut, particularly for pets that are active at night and can't sleep – even if they have been well exercised during the day.
Heather – for pets that constantly want attention.
Impatiens – constant emotional and physical activity, always on the go, never rests for long. May prefer to eat little and often, to restore the energy lost during the day.

CRYSTAL AND GEM ESSENCES
Stibnite – for pets that can never keep still and concentrate, always doing something, never playing with one toy for long. Easily distracted.

HOMEOPATHY
Phosphorus – for thin, nervous hyperactive dogs – especially with a fear of thunder and sudden noises.
Belladonna – for excitability (often with aggressive tendencies).
Coffea – for sleeplessness. Homeopathic coffea will relieve the symptoms that "real" coffee causes.
Scutellaria for hysteria and excitability in general.
Tarentula – odd behavior patterns; dogs, for instance, will catch or chase "imaginary" flies.

HERBAL
Skullcap with **valerian** – the classic calming remedy for the hyperactive pet, especially pets that are destructive when left alone, or always seem on the go, or cannot sleep at night.
Hops are calming and quieting for "manic" behavior in pets

CAUSES

- stress
- food additives
- high levels of dietary protein
- genetic make-up

SIGNS AND SYMPTOMS

- persistent wakefulness
- repetitive behavior
- manic activity

Valerian combined with skullcap is an extremely effective treatment for hyperactivity.

Depression

CAUSES

- physical illness
- stress
- major life event, eg. moving home

SIGNS AND SYMPTOMS

- lethargy
- low energy levels

Pets, like humans, can become depressed and have low energy levels very easily. There are many possible reasons: physical illness can have adverse effects on mental well-being – particularly long-term, chronic illness. Stress, caused by poor housing, insufficient exercise, inadequate diet, overcrowding – or simply living in a household where there is tension and stress within the family – can have depressive effects. Major life events, such as a move of home, the introduction of a new pet (or a new baby), or the death of a close companion (animal or human) can also cause depression.

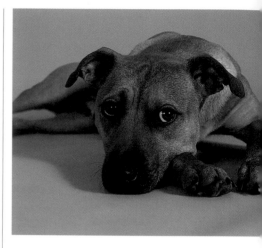

Pets can become depressed as the result of a variety of causes ranging from ill-health to stress.

REMEDIES

AROMATHERAPY
Angelica root – restores and revitalizes pets with low energy levels.
Cedarwood – revives and uplifts when the atmosphere around is tense and stressed.
Citronella – stimulates the nervous system when there is loss of energy.
Lavender – for depression, stress, and difficulty in sleeping.

FLOWER AND GEM REMEDIES
Agrimony – for pets upset by arguments and quarrels around them.
Centaury – when dominated by other animals, very anxious to please.
Cerato – for lack of confidence, always needing reassurance.
Clematis – living in a dream world, inactive, lacking in energy.
Elm – a temporary depression, suddenly overwhelmed by life, in pets that are normally bright and bubbly.
Gentian – easily discouraged, little things are upsetting: a new feeding dish will put them off eating, or a few drops of rain from going for a walk.
Gorse – when willpower is lost in chronic illness, appetite is poor, bowels stop working – everything is "grinding to a halt".

Honeysuckle – for homesickness, depression in boarding kennels or a new home.
Hornbeam – depression and lack of energy at the start of the day, or in chronic illness.
Mustard – intermittent spells of depression, up one day, down the next.
Olive – "post–viral" weakness and depression – after any acute or long-term illness.
Red chestnut – worried and depressed by illness around them.
Star of Bethlehem – for grief, loss, and bereavement.
Sweet chestnut – "end of the tether" feeling, just can't cope any more.
Waratah – depressed by bereavement, or being in kennels.
Bluebell – depressed by bad experiences (abuse or deprivation).
Borage – depressed, elderly or chronically ill pets.
Cucumber – depression and lack of willpower.

Cucumber flower remedy is good for depression.

HERBAL
Ginkgo – tonic for senile, depressed pets.
St Johns Wort – a classic herbal antidepressant. Often known as the herbal "Prozac" – for depression of all kinds.
Damiana – depression, post-viral syndrome, poor appetite.

HOMEOPATHY
Ignatia – for grief, bereavement, all loss.
Gelsemium – weak and depressed, post-viral syndrome.
Opium – lethargy, depression, weakness.

CRYSTAL AND GEM ESSENCES
Chrysophrase – giving in to illness, stimulates willpower.
Herkimer diamond – energizing for dull, depressed pets.
Kyanite – to restore confidence in pets arriving from rescue centers.
Obsidian – improves appetite and energy after loss of a loved companion.
Sardonyx – avoids depression when moving home, or going to a new owner.
Smoky quartz – for any negative state, including depression.

Inappropriate toileting

Leaving urine or feces in unwanted places in the home in the adult animal is usually a behavioral problem rather than a physical disease. In all pets – especially older animals – it is important to check for any possible physical causes. Cystitis, bladder stones, prostate or kidney disease, and urinary incontinence can cause bladder "leakage" around the home. Bowel disease, prostate disease, and CDRM or other nerve diseases can cause loss of fecal control.

If not physical disease, then stress is the likeliest cause of inappropriate toileting. Stressed cats often spray urine, or "midden" (defecate in undesirable places).

REMEDIES

Remedies for anxiety and nervousness (pages 170–171) will be beneficial, and also for hyperactivity (page 173) for those cats that become frantic and cannot rest when under stress. Specific remedies for inappropriate toileting are:

HOMEOPATHY
Staphisagria – where resentment of a new arrival seems the main factor.
Ustillago – especially for male cats spraying urine to mark territory when other male cats are around.
Sepia – for the moody, miserable pet, especially females, that almost seem to be doing it to spite you.

FLOWER AND GEM REMEDIES
Willow for a feeling of resentment.
Impatiens for irritability and impatience with a situation.

CAUSES

- cystitis
- bladder stones
- prostate or kidney disease
- urinary incontinence
- bowel disease

SIGNS AND SYMPTOMS

- spraying urine
- defecating in the home

A litter tray may help with the problem of inappropriate toileting.

Eating disorders

Some pets will stop eating, or need to be coaxed to eat when unwell or stressed. Cats are especially good at driving their owners to distraction by eating one food for a few days, then going on "hunger strike" until something completely different is provided – which is rejected a few days later. This normally seems to be a behavioral trait in cats, and occasionally in dogs and other pets, but is not true anorexia. The most common eating disorder in pets is pica – eating indigestible materials. This can, of course, happen accidentally – dogs that are scavengers, or hamsters eating inappropriate bedding material. The "specialists" for pica are cats.

REMEDIES

If the loss of appetite seems associated with anxiety or depression, use remedies for these problems. General appetite stimulants include **royal jelly, ginseng, and ginkgo.** Treat pica with the following:

AROMATHERAPY
Eucalyptus – to treat the fabric, not the pet; one or two drops on each item discourages.

HOMEOPATHY
Calc. carb. – usually minimizes pica.

FLOWER AND GEM REMEDIES
Wild rose – if pica is a result of boredom.
Chicory – if pica occurs when pet is alone.

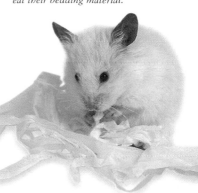

Hamsters sometimes eat their bedding material.

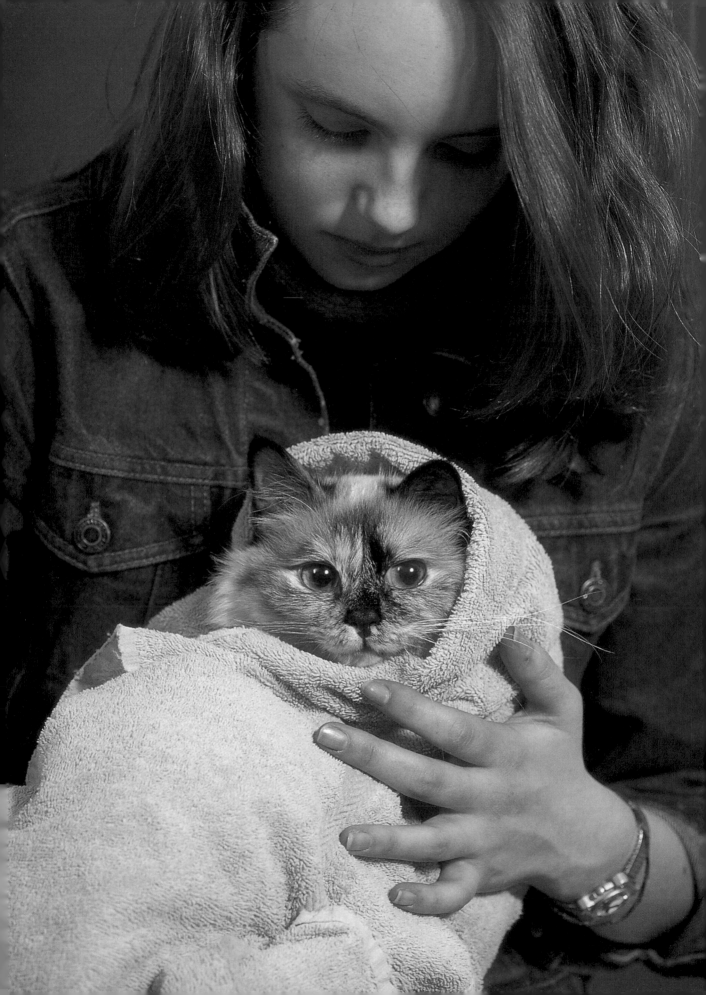

Part IV

In Conclusion:

First Aid and Emergencies

Natural medicines can play an integral role in first aid, but physical first aid and the other measures described here may be required initially. In case surgery is required, do not give an injured pet anything to eat or drink, except on veterinary advice.

ASSESS THE SITUATION

Check whether the injured pet is conscious, breathing, and has a heartbeat.

PREVENT MORE HARM

For example, if the pet has been electrocuted, turn off the power supply immediately, before handling the patient.

CONTACT A VETERINARIAN

Carry out any necessary life-saving procedures, then contact a veterinarian as soon as possible.

RESTRAIN THE PET

Handle all injured pets carefully. If internal injuries are not suspected, wrap small pets in a towel or blanket; alternatively, keep them covered. For dogs, have a muzzle available. Until the pet is moved, cover with a blanket or aluminum foil, to prevent heat loss. This does not, of course, apply if the cause of collapse is heat stroke.

ABOVE *Handle injured pets carefully. Hold them securely and give reassurance.*

CHECK FOR CONSCIOUSNESS

1 A conscious pet will react to a sudden noise (for example, clapping by their ears), to pinching of the skin between the toes, or by blinking if a hand is passed in front of his or her eyes.

2 To check for breathing, watch the chest closely to see whether it is rising and falling, bend down and listen carefully, or hold a feather in front of the pet's nose and watch for movement.

3 To feel for a heartbeat, press your fingers firmly against the chest.

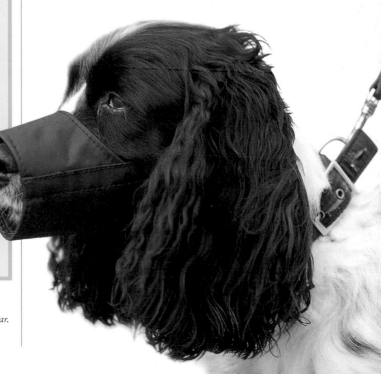

LEFT *Small animals and cats can be wrapped in a blanket for warmth and security while waiting for treatment.*

RIGHT *An injured dog may snap or bite due to pain or fear. Use a muzzle until the dog is secure and comfortable.*

Basic first aid

CLEAR THE AIRWAY

If the pet is not breathing, or is choking, check for obstructions to the airway. With the pet on its side, open the jaws and gently pull the tongue forward. Remove any debris in the nose, mouth, or throat.

ARTIFICIAL RESPIRATION

If the pet is not breathing but there is a heartbeat, breathing may be restored with artificial respiration.

Close the pet's mouth and, keeping it closed, gently blow directly into the nostrils until you see the chest rise. Then let the lungs deflate naturally before beginning the process again. Repeat this procedure 15 times per minute, or until breathing starts spontaneously. Keep checking the chest for signs of breathing by bending down and listening closely, or by watching to see if the chest moves.

HEART MASSAGE

If there is no breathing or heartbeat, alternate 15-second spells of artificial respiration with 15-second periods of heart massage. To do this, use the fingers and thumb of one hand to squeeze the chest wall, compress the

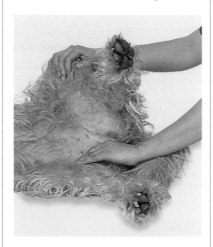

Before starting artificial respiration, or heart massage, check to see if there is a pulse and listen for breathing.

chest strongly, then release. Repeat as frequently as possible (at least once, or preferably twice per second). Alternate heart massage with artificial respiration until the heart restarts, and then continue with artificial respiration until breathing starts.

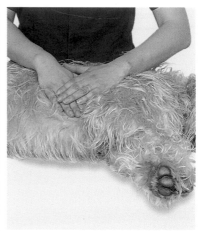

Massage the heart by compressing the chest wall firmly and rhythmically once or twice per second until the heartbeat returns.

CONTROL BLEEDING

If a wound is bleeding uncontrollably, apply pressure at the point of bleeding. Any padding is suitable. Apply absorbent padding, overlaid by as many layers of firm bandaging material as necessary, until the bleeding stops.

If an object is protruding from the wound, do not try to pull it out as you may cause more damage. Make a ring-shaped pad by twisting a length of material into a donut shape and place this around the wound before gently bandaging the pad in position.

Bandage a wound only if the bleeding is severe. You should not apply a tourniquet above the bleeding point: this can obstruct the blood supply to healthy tissue and cause permanent damage. Raising the pet's hindquarters will assist the blood flow to the heart and head.

〇 *Make a ring-shaped pad by taking a length of cotton wool or bandaging and twisting it into a circular shape.*

〇 *Wrap narrow gauze around the ring to retain the shape and give some rigidity.*

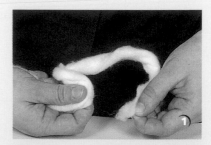

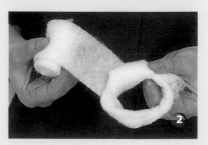

Wounds

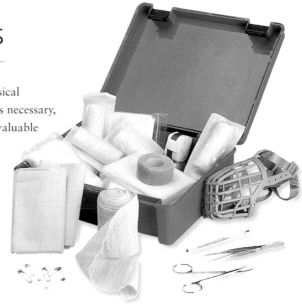

Carry out any physical first–aid measures necessary, then make use of the valuable assistance of natural medicines.

A well-equipped first–aid kit for pets is invaluable, as human first–aid kits will be inadequate for the needs of animals.

PREVENTION

Prevention is better than cure.

• Ensure dogs are well-trained and obedient. Concentrate on teaching them to come when called and to be well behaved near traffic.

• Keep all household cleaners, medicines, and poisonous plants out of the reach. If your pet is a "nibbler," keep all electrical cords out of reach.

• Ensure cages and tanks have no projections that can cause injuries.

• Avoid outdoor danger. Don't leave pets in cars on warm days. Don't let dogs hold their heads out of car windows. Don't let dogs chase sheep. Keep safely and securely stored and labeled all garden and garage chemicals.

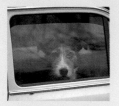

Pets should not be left in cars on hot days.

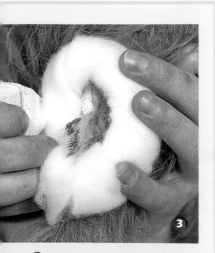

Place the ring bandage around the protrusion and carefully bandage it in place. Make sure that the protruding object is not pressed by any bandaging.

REMEDIES

AROMATHERAPY

Tea tree (diluted) can be applied directly to wounds to clean and act as an antiseptic.

Geranium – stimulates healing of wound.

Lavender – relieves pain and prompts healing. Lavender can safely be applied neat to a wound.

Camomile (German and Roman) reduces the inflammation and pain of recent wounds.

Clove bud – good for cuts and ulcerated wounds.

Thyme is excellent for cuts and bruises.

Vetivert is a good wound healer, and also calms and relieves shock.

Yarrow helps heal cuts and wounds, and is a revitalizing remedy for those pets feeling down and depressed after their wound. Only **lavender** and **tea tree** should be applied directly to the wound. The other oils should be massaged around the wound, or used by diffusion (see pages 28–29).

HERBAL

A **witch hazel** compress will help reduce swelling and bruising.

Marigold tincture applied to the wound will prevent infection and promote healing. Tincture of **myrrh** is a good antiseptic, and can be put into any bandage used to dress the wound.

Geranium leaves can be wrapped round the wound, and kept in place with strips of medical tape (do not tape on too tightly).

HOMEOPATHY

Arnica – reduces bruising, stops bleeding, and accelerates healing.

Calendula – apply calendula tincture or cream directly to the wound to stimulate healing.

Ledum and **Hypericum** – for puncture wounds. **Ledum** helps prevent tetanus, **Hypericum** – minimizes pain and discomfort.

Hepar. sulph. – if wound is infected.

NUTRITIONAL

Honey or **sugar** smeared on the wound will promote healing, and reduce the risk of scarring.

FLOWER AND GEM REMEDIES

Rescue Remedy can be applied directly to the wound – but dilute as the alcohol base may sting.

Almond – rejuvenates and heals damaged tissue.

Mango also speeds healing after injuries.

Almonds

Bites and stings

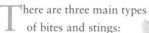

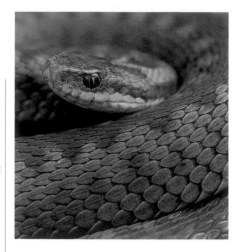

There are three main types of bites and stings:
- Animal;
- Insect;
- Poisonous snakes, insects, and jellyfish.

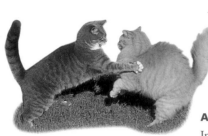

Fighting cats can cause quite severe wounds.

Adder bites and bee stings cause localized pain with itching and swelling and sometimes allergic reaction. Homeopathic treatments are effective.

ANIMAL BITES

In the case of animal bites, treat as for wounds (see page 179). For cat bites that leave puncture wounds, always use homeopathic Ledum and Hypericum.

INSECT STINGS

Bees, wasps, and other insect bites and stings usually cause local pain, itching, and swelling at the site of the sting. Occasionally a severe allergic reaction occurs, leading to collapse and shock (see below). For local reactions, treatment with natural medicines is very effective.

DOS AND DON'TS

Suspected poisonous bites are obviously an emergency and need immediate veterinary treatment.

Never try to suck the poison from such a bite – it increases the blood supply to the area and increases the risk. Use an ice pack on the bite to reduce blood supply.

For jellyfish stings, look for and remove any remaining tentacles (but wear gloves).

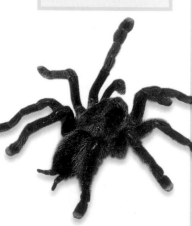

Tarentula remedy is proven from the infamous tarantula spider.

REMEDIES

AROMATHERAPY
Neat **lavender** applied to the sting will relieve swelling and discomfort.
Tea tree oil applied directly will reduce the possibility of infection.
Geranium (diluted) will encourage healing. Essential oils can be used as insect repellents to reduce the likelihood of insect stings. Dilute a few drops of **citronella, lemon eucalyptus,** and **cinnamon leaf** in 1 cup (300 ml) of water, and comb this through the fur. Repeat daily.

FLOWER AND GEM REMEDIES
Rescue Remedy is available as a cream, which can be applied directly to the sting.

HERBAL
Witch hazel applied to stings will cool and soothe.
Marigold tincture will reduce the reaction to bee stings.

NUTRITIONAL
Cucumber juice and **scallion juice** will relieve soreness and discomfort.

HOMEOPATHY
Apis. mel. – ideal for the swelling and irritation of insect stings.
Cantharis – for acute burning pain and redness.
Hypericum – for the pain and soreness.
Urtica – for the itchiness following a sting.
Vespa – specific for wasp stings.

OTHERS
Apply an ice pack to reduce inflammation. Bites from poisonous snakes and spiders give symptoms of drooling, trembling, and rapid collapse and shock (see below). Jellyfish stings cause pain, agitation, and restlessness. Treat as for stings (above).
Additional remedies include:

HOMEOPATHY
Cedron and **echinacea** will help reduce toxic effect of poisons.
Elaps, lachesis, and **crotalus horridus** are homeopathic remedies made from snake venoms, which will be helpful, depending on the symptoms, for the later reaction to snake bites.
Tarentula is a remedy from the poisonous spider – useful for the reaction to spider poisons.

Hemorrhage

Externally this varies from simple oozing from a graze or laceration, to spurting blood when an artery has been cut, perhaps after a road traffic accident. Internal bleeding is less obvious. The pet will have pale or white gums and be breathing rapidly, but the breathing may be shallow, will be weak, and the animal may collapse. Extremities such as feet and ears will feel cool to the touch.

Internal bleeding may be the result of accidents or injuries, caused by infection such as hepatitis follow poisoning, or be the result of clotting defects, such as hemophilia (see Anemia, page 100).

Pets may suffer hemorrhage as a complication after giving birth.

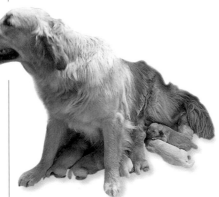

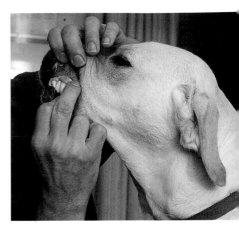

ABOVE *Check for pale gums and rapid breathing if internal bleeding is suspected.*

REMEDIES

To treat a hemorrhage, carry out any necessary physical first–aid measures, concentrating on the measures to control bleeding. Use the remedies for collapse and shock if necessary. **Vitamin K** is a specific antidote to warfarin poisoning, but will need to be given at your veterinary practice by injection. Blood transfusion may be necessary for severe hemorrhage.

AROMATHERAPY
Lavender massaged around the site of the hemorrhage will reduce bruising and swelling.

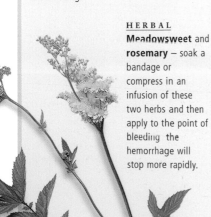

HERBAL
Meadowsweet and **rosemary** – soak a bandage or compress in an infusion of these two herbs and then apply to the point of bleeding the hemorrhage will stop more rapidly.

Meadowsweet can be used with rosemany to stop hemorrhage.

HOMEOPATHY
Arnica – the greatest of all remedies for tissue damage and hemorrhage following injuries. Minimizes bruising. Give as a preventative before operations or dental treatment to reduce the risk of bleeding.
Aconite – use if the blood is bright red. Especially good for nosebleeds and any situation where there is bleeding with shock. Good for bleeding after operations.
Ipecac – use if the blood is bright red. Useful for blood being passed in milk from nursing animals and for severe bleeding accompanied by heavy breathing.
Phosphorus – for watery, bright blood. Especially useful for persistent bleeding and wounds that won't stop oozing blood.
Hamamelis – dark, seeping blood. Particularly good to absorb the blood from aural hematomas (see page 78) and bleeding inside eyes.
Millefolium – use if the blood is bright red, often hemorrhaging from several different points. Useful to treat warfarin poisoning.

Lachesis – dark, purplish bleeding from septic wounds. Blood does not clot easily. Useful after snake bites.
Kreosotum – hemorrhage from small ulcerated wounds, and around infected decaying teeth and gums.
Acid nit. – bleeding from warts, and from ulceration around nostrils and in gums.
Sabina – especially for bright red hemorrhage from the uterus, usually after giving birth.

FLOWER AND GEM REMEDIES
Rescue Remedy should be given by mouth to minimize the shock when there is severe bleeding following accidents or injuries.

CRYSTAL AND GEM ESSENCES
Carnelion, hematite, and **ruby** will all slow down bleeding and improve clotting. They are particularly useful for persistent bleeding, and for internal hemorrhage.

NUTRITIONAL
Powdered eggshells applied to a bleeding point will promote rapid clotting.
Baked, dried chicken also has a clotting effect when applied to bleeding joints.

Collapse and shock

CAUSES

- poisoning
- heart disease
- obstruction in throat
- diabetes
- convulsions
- disc protrusion
- poisoning bites
- electrocution
- eclampsia
- anaphylactic shock

SIGNS AND SYMPTOMS

- **early symptoms:** increased breathing and heart rate; paler gums than normal; restlessness and anxiety; body feeling cooler; weakness
- **later symptoms:** shallow, slow breathing; irregular, slow heartbeat; white or blue gums; extreme weakness or unconsciousness; body is cold to touch

Sudden collapse and shock can be caused by an enormous variety of conditions: The early symptoms of shock are increased breathing and heart rate, paler gums than normal, restlessness and anxiety, body feeling slightly cooler, and weakness. Later symptoms include shallow, slow breathing, irregular and slow heartbeat, white or blue gums, extreme weakness and lethargy or unconsciousness, and a body temperature that is cold to the touch.

Obstruction by objects in the throat can cause sudden collapse.

REMEDIES

Treat with the first aid measures given above and following:
- Place the pet on its side, with the head extended – this helps normal breathing.
- Raise the hindquarters – this increases blood flow to the heart and brain.
- Wrap in a warm covering, or aluminum foil to preserve body heat.
- Treat any obvious injuries or bleeding with remedies described above.
- Get veterinary attention immediately.
- While waiting for veterinary attention, the following natural remedies may be life-saving:

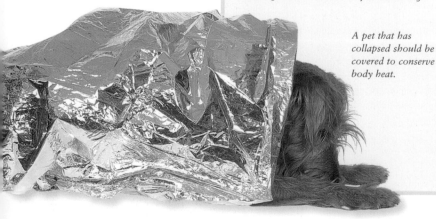

A pet that has collapsed should be covered to conserve body heat.

AROMATHERAPY
Melissa – minimizes shock and trauma.

FLOWER AND GEM REMEDIES
Rescue Remedy – for all types of collapse and shock.
An essential remedy at this time. Can be given to unconscious patients.

HOMEOPATHY
Aconite – for conscious or unconscious patients.
Carbo veg. – for the weak, collapsed pet with a desire for fresh air.
Veratrum alb. – collapse, blue gums, often with diarrhea.
Arnica – for collapse with physical injuries.
Pyrogen – weak, high temperature, collapse caused by acute infection and fever.
Camphor – icy coldness, often with dilated staring pupils and black diarrhea.

Poisoning

Apart from poisonous bites and stings (see page 180), poisoning can occur in three ways: skin contact, inhaled, or swallowed.

SKIN CONTACT POISONING

With skin contact poisoning, skin damage and burns can be caused by paint, paint stripper, motor oil, tar and other petroleum products, and many other chemicals. The mouth may also be burned if the skin is licked. Stinging nettles can also cause severe reaction in short-haired pets.

To treat paint, tar, and petroleum product poisoning, wear rubber gloves and rub large amounts of vegetable or mineral oil into the affected area, then wash with plenty of warm, soapy water. Rinse well, and repeat till all traces are removed. Mild detergents may be used as cleansing agents. Do not use turpentine or methylated spirit to clean the area.

With other products, wash the affected area with clean, cool water for 3 minutes, then wash with warm soapy water, rinse, and repeat till clear. Mild detergents may be used as cleansing agents.

In the case of stinging nettles, wash with cool, clean water. Keep the pet active and alert to help stop shock developing. Give homeopathic Urtica – a specific antidote. In all cases, treat as for collapse and shock if appropriate, and give general poison remedies (see page 185).

INHALED POISONS

Inhaled poisons (smoke and fumes during fires, insecticidal sprays, and fumes from non stick utensils) can all be damaging. They affect breathing, and may cause neurological symptoms.

Pets that groom themselves may ingest chemicals on their coat.

SKIN POISONING

CAUSES

- petroleum products or other chemicals
- stinging nettles

SIGNS AND SYMPTOMS

- skin damage and burns

INHALED POISONS

CAUSES

- smoke and fumes during fires
- insecticidal sprays
- fumes from nonstick utensils

SIGNS AND SYMPTOMS

- breathing difficulties
- neurological problems

POISONS: EMERGENCY ACTION

Treat for collapse and shock (see above) and give any physical first-aid measures necessary.
- If poison has been swallowed in the last two hours, the pet is conscious and alert, and the poison is not acid, alkali, or petroleum-based, make the pet vomit. Use a large crystal of washing soda (sodium carbonate) or a concentrated salt solution, giving every 10 minutes until vomiting occurs.
- Do not try to make unconscious pets or pets (other than cats and dogs) vomit.
- Give activated charcoal if available – 1–2 teaspoons. This absorbs ingested poisons.
- If the poison is known, your veterinarian will have access to a poisons information center for specific advice on treatment.
- If the poison is not known, keep for analysis any evidence – remains of poison, labels, boxes, even any vomit brought up.

- If the poison is acid/alkali or petroleum-based do not make your pet vomit. For acid poisons, give baking soda, bicarbonate of soda, egg white or olive oil by mouth (if the patient is conscious) and apply baking soda to any mouth burns. For alkali poisons, give egg white, small amounts of vinegar or citrus fruit juice by mouth (if the patient is conscious), and apply vinegar to mouth burns. Most household products will have an acid or alkali symbol on the labels.

INHALED POISONS

Treat as for collapse and shock and give general poison remedies.

Cats are renown for prowling around the home or garden, so keep all chemical products out of reach.

CAUSES

- acids, alkalis, and petroleum products in home or general environment
- drugs
- poisonous plants

SIGNS AND SYMPTOMS

- vomiting
- diarrhea
- shock
- burns to skin or mouth
- **insecticidal poisoning:** twitching, trembling, salivation
- **rodent poisons:** internal bleeding
- **antifreeze:** wobbling, vomiting, and convulsions

EMERGENCY ACTION

In all cases of poisoning – even if there is a specific natural antidote – immediate veterinary attention is required.

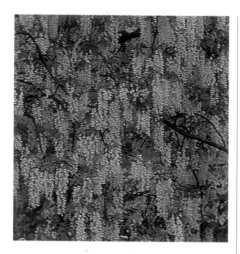

Laburnum seeds are highly poisonous to all animals.

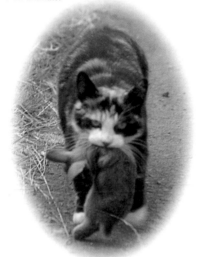

Catching poisoned rodents can be equally dangerous to pets.

SWALLOWED POISONS

Swallowed poisons can be found in and around the home. Among the most common are:

- Acids, alkalis, and petroleum products (caustic soda, chlorine bleach and tablets) and other products (insecticidal shampoos, collars and sprays, slug and snail baits, etc.).
- Drugs – aspirin, human prescription drugs (sedatives and antidepressants), illegal drugs (cannabis, ecstasy, and others).

- Poisonous plants, trees, and shrubs (for example, all flower bulbs, horse chestnut, and yew).

Most poisons cause broadly similar symptoms – vomiting, diarrhea, shock, burns to skin or mouth. Insecticidal poisoning causes nervous symptoms – twitching, trembling, salivation. Some rodent poisons cause internal bleeding; some cause stiffness and convulsions; some cause initial hyperactivity, later sedation and hypothermia. Slug bait poisoning causes tremors, salivation, and convulsions.

Antifreeze (ethylene glycol) causes wobbling, vomiting and convulsions. Aspirin poisoning leads to poor appetite, depression, abdominal pain, uncoordination. Aspirin in small amounts is safe for most dogs, and low doses are sometimes prescribed for cats, but large amounts are poisonous, and cats are particularly sensitive to aspirin. Aspirin is poisonous to smaller pets even in minute quantities.

- Illegal drugs mostly cause uncoordination, restlessness, dilated pupils, anxiety and sometimes biting from fear. Animals don't usually seem to experience any of the "highs" of drugs that humans do. Keep affected pets in dark, quiet surroundings. Homeopathic Cannabis is a specific antidote to cannabis poisoning.
- Prescription drugs that have toxic effects are usually sedatives or antidepressants, so effects are either uncoordination and sedation, or alternatively restlessness and rapid heart-beat.
- Lead poisoning causes vomiting and diarrhoea, later anxiety, staggering, paralysis, and dislike of light. The homeopathic remedy Plumbum met. is a specific antidote to lead poisoning and should be given as soon as possible.

REMEDIES : EMERGENCY TREATMENT

Apart from physical first–aid measures, and treatment for collapse and shock, the following natural remedies will help poison victims:

AROMATHERAPY
Lavender will aid recovery from poisoning.

HOMOEOPATHY
Nux vomica – will help neutralize the effect of all poisons, especially poisonous plants and strychnine-based poisons.
Arsen. alb. – for all cases where vomiting and diarrhea are the main symptoms.
Opium – for weakness, paralysis, coma, heavy breathing, twitching muscles.
Phosphorus – vomiting with blood, lung damage (including coughing up blood), liver damage.
Stramonium – for poisons causing staggering, falling forward, dilated pupils, twitching of muscles and fits.

Strychninum – for strychnine poisoning, and other poisons causing similar symptoms.
Agaricus – follows a pattern of initially slight stimulation and excitability, followed by uncoordination with twitching and noticeable over-reaction to light and noise, followed by great excitability, often with crying out and screaming, followed by depression, sedation, and coma. This remedy will treat alphachloralose poisoning, and other poisons causing similar symptoms.
Apomorphine – for poison causing repeated, painful vomiting. Do not use this remedy if you are trying to make your pet vomit.
Belladonna – for poisons causing fever, restlessness, dilated pupils, sore mouth and excessive thirst, hysteria and fits.
Zinc – uncoordination with a tendency to fall to the left, trembling and twitching of muscles, blisters on tongue and gums.
Scutellaria – for poisons causing great excitability and hysteria, and later convulsions.

REMEDIES : RECOVERY TREATMENT

Animals being treated for poisoning; which are beginning to recover, will benefit from the following remedies to strengthen them and help remove the damage the poison has caused:

FLOWER AND GEM REMEDIES
Hornbeam – is strengthening and aids convalescence after poisoning.
Crab apple – a cleansing agent, helps remove toxins of all kinds from the body.
Gorse – for pets weakened and losing the will to live.
Olive – a "tonic" for lethargy and weakness following poisoning.
Camphor – a cleansing, detoxifying agent.
Zucchini – a convalescent remedy, builds up strength.

HERBAL
Elderberry – a blood purifier, removes toxins from the bloodstream.

Yellow dock – a liver support remedy, to improve detoxification of poisons.

CRYSTAL AND GEM ESSENCES
Clear quartz – keep near the affected pet when ill to cleanse and detoxify the body.
Labradorite – to improve will power and promote healing.

HOMEOPATHY
China and **Phos. acid** – both help restore health and strength in debilitated animals after poisoning.
Kali. carb. – good for pets weakened by liver or kidney damage after being poisoned.

Gorse will strengthen pets that are giving up.

DOS AND DON'TS

Prevention is always better than cure, so ensure that you keep all prescription medicines and cleaning and garden materials locked away in cabinets.

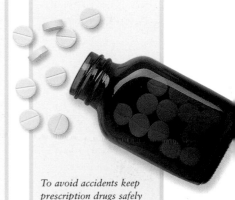

To avoid accidents keep prescription drugs safely out of reach from pets.

Do not use weedkillers or rodent poisons in areas to which pets have access. Ensure all containers of medicines, chemicals, or any products are clearly and carefully labeled so that if an incident does occur the name of the product will be known.

Burns and scalds

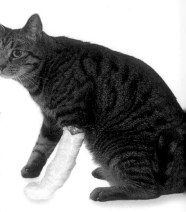

Most burns are caused by fire, heat, or hot liquids. Chemicals can also cause caustic burns, and pets that chew electrical wires can receive electrical burns. Sunburn is another possible cause.

To treat any of the above:
• Do not spread butter or fats on burns.
• If a burn is from a caustic chemical, wear rubber gloves to avoid hurting yourself.

• When a burn is electrical, switch off power before touching the pet.
• Veterinary treatment is essential for all burns, except very minor superficial wounds.
• Flush the burned area with cool water, and apply an ice pack as soon as possible to reduce pain and inflammation. Keep the ice pack in place for 15 minutes.

All burns need veterinary attention in order for the damaged area to be correctly sterilized and bandaged.

REMEDIES

AROMATHERAPY
Lavender and **rosemary** massaged around the burn will be soothing and healing.
Geranium – a few drops per 4 cups (1 liter) should be added to the cool water used to bathe the burn. It will encourage healing.

HERBAL
Aloe vera can be applied once the burn has been cooled to promote healing.
Echinacea – a few drops in 2 cups (500 ml) water applied to the burn will help keep infection out.

HOMEOPATHY
Cantharis – ideal to relieve the pain of burns and scalds, reduce inflammation, and let healing take place.

Urtica – will help relieve the itching as the burn begins to heal.
Arnica – will reduce skin trauma from burns.

NUTRITIONAL
A **raw potato** placed on the burn gives instant short-term relief.
Honey applied to the burn will speed up healing and keep infection out.

Heat stroke

SIGNS AND SYMPTOMS

• panting
• salivating
• disorientation
• collapse

This is seen as panting, salivating, disorientation, and collapse.

Remove the pet from the heat; immerse in a cool bath or spray with cool water.

Place an ice pack on the head to reduce heat to the brain. Give cold water to drink. In severe cases treat for collapse and shock (see page 182) and get veterinary attention.

REMEDIES

AROMATHERAPY
Camomile (Roman) – soothes and calms.

FLOWER AND GEM REMEDIES
Mulla mulla and **sunflower** can both be used to treat and to help prevent heatstroke.

HOMEOPATHY
Belladonna and **Glonoine** both help bring down body temperature rapidly.

A pet suffering from heat should be cooled with water and an ice pack to the head.

PAIN REMEDIES

Natural medicines are effective against most kinds of pain.

AROMATHERAPY
Celery seed for neuritis and all nerve pains.
German camomile for teething pains and painful joints.

FLOWER AND GEM REMEDIES
Sapphire – for back pain and neuritis.
Avocado – for "growing pains" in young animals.
St. John's Wort – a general painkiller.

HERBAL
Yarrow for aches and pains in joints.
Camomile for teething pains in young pets.
St John's wort for chronic back pain and neuritis.
White willow for back, joint, and muscle pain.
Feverfew for arthritic pain.

CRYSTAL AND GEM ESSENCES
Amber – for stomach pains and toothache.
Blue lace agate for pain of arthritis.
Coral – general aches and pains, especially abdominal.
Jet for toothache and pains in the head.
Lapis lazuli – for all pain, especially in head, eyes, or ears.
Reticulated quartz for muscle, joint and back pain, and pain of insect bites.
Sapphire for pain from slipped discs and trapped nerves.

HOMEOPATHY
Acid sal. – pain in small joints.
Camomile – teething pains.
Causticum – joint pains in stiff, old pets.
Hepar. sulph. – pain from abscesses.
Hypericum – pain from damaged nerves, slipped discs, all spinal problems, and post-operative pain.
Ledum – pain from puncture wounds.
Mag. phos. – muscle cramps and pains.

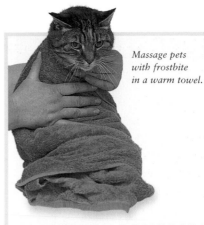

Massage pets with frostbite in a warm towel.

FROSTBITE REMEDIES

The extremities – tops of ears, tail, and feet – are most likely to be affected by frostbite. Massage the affected area gently with a warm towel or in lukewarm water (not hot). If the skin darkens, get veterinary treatment urgently.

HOMEOPATHY
Agaricus – helps frost-bitten tissues recover.
Arnica – heals all damaged tissue.
AROMATHERAPY
Lavender can be applied directly to damaged area to promote healing.

TRAVEL SICKNESS REMEDIES

It is possible to give human travel sickness tablets to pets, in small doses, but effects are very variable, and often leave the pet drowsy for a while at the end of the journey. Conventional veterinary treatment has the same effect of sedation, but leaves a very wobbly pet at journey's end.

With natural medicine, pets that are anxious and nervous in cars or other methods of transport, as opposed to being truly "travel sick," should be given remedies for nervousness and anxiety (see page 170). For true motion sickness – which may include a degree of anxiety too – use the following:

HERBAL
Angelica leaves – hang in the car while traveling.
Peppermint – give your pet peppermint tea before a journey.
Fennel or **camomile** tea will also ease symptoms.

AROMATHERAPY
Ginger – massaged or used by diffuser before a journey, is very effective.

NUTRITIONAL
Ginger – if there isn't time to use essential oil of ginger, give a little "real" ginger by mouth. If you don't have any, a ginger biscuit will do!

HOMEOPATHY
Petroleum – very effective in most cases.
Diesel smoke – self–evidently used for diesel–engined cars, to good effect.
Tabacum – especially good for sea sickness.
Cocculus – another classic, effective antisickness remedy.

FLOWER AND GEM REMEDIES
Scleranthus for motion sickness.
Sweet flag and **sweet chestnut** for dislike of being in a car.

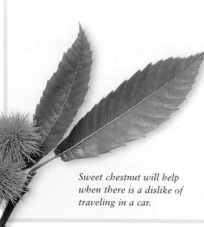

Sweet chestnut will help when there is a dislike of traveling in a car.

Feed your pet ginger biscuits mixed with their normal food, to help prevent travel sickness.

Saying Goodbye

However healthy a pet has been throughout life, the fact remains that all pets live far shorter lives than we do – with the possible exception of tortoises! At some point, natural lifespan comes to an end. We all hope that when our pets die they will pass away naturally in their sleep. However, if a pet is in severe pain or is terminally ill, the choice has to be made sometimes to carry out euthanasia.

MAKING THE DECISION

Before that point is reached, it is important for peace of mind, that everything possible has been done for the pet concerned. It is all too difficult in an old, arthritic pet, with failing liver and kidneys, to decide when the line has been crossed beyond which quality of life is too poor to continue.

In these circumstances, veterinary advice is vital. But once you are satisfied there is nothing more that can help your pet, you have to make the decision.

There are no "natural ways" of performing euthanasia. However, there are natural remedies that can help to make the last few days or weeks of life as comfortable and enjoyable as possible. Natural medicines for pain may be appropriate, and remedies for specific conditions such as cancer, arthritis, kidney disease, and so on will be essential. Natural treatments for these diseases not only help to slow down deterioration of the condition, but also ensure the pet being treated feels as well as possible.

If euthanasia has to be performed, then natural remedies for anxiety and nervousness can be used beforehand to keep the pet as calm as possible. It may also be appropriate to give conventional sedatives or tranquilizers.

Euthanasia is the final positive step you can take on behalf of your pet. It is important to remember it is a positive act, not a negative one. You are preventing pain, suffering, and an undignified end to life. Having done all you can for your pet throughout life, you need to do all you can at the end of life, to make it a smooth, gentle transition from life to death.

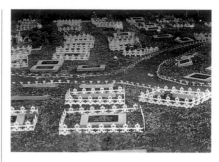

There are several options available when your pet has died, including burial in a pet cemetary. Your veterinarian can offer advice.

PLANNING AHEAD

Planning beforehand is essential. Do you want the euthanasia carried out at home? Do you want to be with your pet, or wait outside? What happens afterward – do you want the ashes back after cremation? Would you prefer a burial? Do you want some kind of memorial, would you consider the services of a taxidermist? Do you want to bury the body in your own garden? Do you want children, or other members of the family present? Although distressing for children, it can be even more distressing for them to arrive home to a fait accompli.

If euthanasia is carried out at the veterinary practice, ask for an appointment away from normal consulting times when you won't have to sit and wait with other people and pets, and won't risk other appointments over-running.

Always have someone with you. Make sure you don't have to drive home alone after such an event. After euthanasia – whether you stayed with your pet or not – always say a proper goodbye. Take as long as you want, and don't be embarrassed about weeping.

For the next few days, make sure you have support. Don't be ashamed or guilty about grieving for a pet. There are pet bereavement counselors or general counselors who can guide and support you through the grieving process.

Finally, think carefully before taking on another pet. Don't rush into it. But equally, don't feel you don't ever want another pet, because you can't replace the one you have lost. Sooner or later, most of us, having said goodbye, will say hello to another pet in need of love, attention – and natural healthcare!

If your pet is in pain or terminally ill, it may be appropriate to consider euthanasia as a positive act.

The Way Forward

In an ideal world, your local veterinary team would be trained and knowledgeable in all aspects of veterinary medicine – including natural therapies for pets.

However, in reality your nearest veterinarian practicing such natural therapies may be some distance away. The aim of this book is to have a reference work to hand, so that for minor ailments your pet can have the benefit of natural therapies; for more serious problems, natural medicines can complement necessary conventional treatment, and if attention is paid to a healthy lifestyle and diet, less treatment of any kind will be required.

A NEW APPROACH

The way forward from now on, for all of us, is to integrate a natural approach to healthcare for our pets into the world at large. It means a concern for the environment, for the quality of our water, our air, and our soil. There is a mass of knowledge and wisdom about natural cures and folk remedies, the cycles of the seasons, the whole relationship between us and the earth on which we live.

We need to take more responsibility for our own health and that of our pets. We need to be able to discuss symptoms, be given options as to investigations and

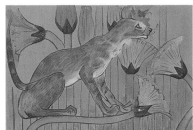

Traditional knowledge of medical treatment and therapy is making a comeback.

treatments, understand how diagnoses are arrived at – in other words, to share in the decision-making process about our pets' health and treatment.

This guide will give you one reference text to draw on. But any single book has its limitations and so this book should be a starting point. There is more information in libraries, in bookstores, and on the internet. There are courses, seminars, and lecture days on natural therapies. There are stores stocking wide ranges of natural medicines from Chinese herbs to homeopathic medicines.

There is a sea change taking place in medicine. The old knowledge is making a comeback, along with new knowledge of the immune system and the functioning of internal body processes. Natural therapies are no longer on the fringe of medicine. They are taking their rightful place as an equal partner to Western conventional medicine in the treatment of disease and the maintenance of health.

Traditional and conventional medicine – the old and the new, ancient and modern. The way forward is to embrace the best of both traditions to give our pets the happiest and healthiest life we possibly can.

Traditional Chinese Medicine and therapies such as acupuncture are now accepted alternatives.

Further Information

The author can be contacted at:

Natural Veterinary Medicine Center
11 Southgate Road
Potters Bar
Hertfordshire
EN6 5DR. UK
Tel: 01707 662058

(The author cannot guarantee a response to all enquiries.)

ORGANIZATIONS

UK
British Society of Homeopathic Veterinary Surgeons (BAHVS)
Chinham House
Stanford-in-the-Vale
Farringdon
Oxfordshire SN7 8NQ
Tel: 01376 710324

Holistic Health Foundation
2 De La Hay Avenue
Plymouth
Devon PL3 4HH
Tel: 01752 671485

National Veterinary Acupuncture Association
85 Earls Court Road
London
W8 6EF
Tel: 0207 9378215

US
Academy of Veterinary Homeopathy
751 N.E. 168th Street
N. Miami Beach
FL 33162-2427
Tel: 305 652 1590
www.acadvetvom.org

American Holistic Veterinary Medical Association
2218 Old Emmorton Road
Bel Air
MD 21015
Tel: 410 569 0795
www.altvetmed.com

International Veterinary Acupuncture Society
2140 Conestoga Road
Chester Springs
PA 19425
Tel: 215 827 7245

SUPPLIERS

UK
Ainsworths Homeopathic Pharmacy
38 New Cavendish Street
London W1M 7LH
Tel: 0207 4955330

Bach Flower Remedies Ltd
Mount Vernon
Sotwell, Wallingford
Oxfordshire OX10 0PZ
Tel: 01491 834678

Denes Natural Pet Care
PO Box 691
2 Osmond Road
Hove BN3 3SD
Tel: 01273 325364

Dorwest Herbs (Veterinary)
Shipton Gorge
Bridport
Dorset DT6 4LP
Tel: 01308 897272

Freeman's Chemist
20 Main Street
Busby

Glasgow G76 8DU
Tel: 0141 6441165
www.freechem.co.uk

US
Boericke and Tafel
2381 Circedian Way
Santa Rosa
CA 95407
Tel: 800 876 9505

Boiron USA
PO Box 449
6 Campus Boulevard
Bldg A
Newtown Square
PA 19073
Tel: 800 253 8823

Ellon (Bach USA) Inc.
PO Box 320
Woodmere
NY 11598
Tel: 516 593 2206

Natural Health Supply
6410 Avenida de Christina
Santa Fe
NM 87505
Tel: 888 689 1608

PICTURE CREDITS AND ACKNOWLEDGMENTS

Bob Langerish: 59tr, 63bc; Bruce Coleman Collection: Gunter Ziesler 22, John Cancalosi 180tr, Animal Ark 173br; David Alderton: 12t, 47tr, 74cl, 75br, 116tr, 166tl, 168cl, 172tl; Dennis Avon: 60r, 73c, 148tr; David English: 54b; David Parker/Science Picture Library: 26t; Garden Picture Library: 48bc, 184t; G. Hadjo, CNRI/Science Picture Library: 56tc; Hahnemann House Trust: 44tl; Image Bank: 52t, 62c, 171tr, 172bl; Jane Burton – Warren Photographic: 12b, 18bl, 56bl, 66, 160, 163r; Mark Jamieson: 11, 64, 65b; Michael Courtney: 57tr, 162c, 164br, 165tc; The Art Archive/Biblioteca Nazionale Marciana Venice/Dagki Orti (A): 41t; The Veterinary Centre: 97tr, 97r, 98t, 99t, 108l, 108r, 114c, 114l, 119tr; Tony Stone: 2, 7, 8, 127tr.
(t=top, b=bottom, l=left, r=right, c=center)

The publishers would like to thank Brian Turner and Simon Scott of The Veterinary Centre, Welwyn Garden City, UK for use of x-ray images, and Mark Jamieson and Michael Courtney for their illustrations. Marc Henrie would like to thank all those who offered their time, material – and pets – to help produce the photography for this book.

Index

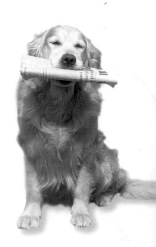